FACE IT!

HARSH SKINCARE
TRUTHS EVERY
ESTHETICIAN
SHOULD KNOW...
AND SO SHOULD YOU

TANIS RHINES, MA, LE
NEDDY RODRIGUEZ, LE, MUA

AUTHOR'S DISCLAIMER

In this book, Ms. Rhines and Ms. Rodriguez offer general advice and their opinions about skincare. Both are estheticians licensed to practice in Florida and California and the information is general in nature. What they say is not a substitute for medical advice from a dermatologist, physician, or other healthcare provider.

Each person's skin and body are different; what works for one person may not achieve good results for you. If you have sensitivity or a reaction to any product or procedure described in this book, then you should stop using it and consult a dermatologist, physician, or other healthcare provider.

With these precautionary measures in mind, the authors ask you to sit back, relax, and enjoy the book. We hope you find the contents informative and entertaining.

In honor of our divine responsibility to the truth.

~ VERITAS AEQUITAS

CONTENTS

INTRODUCTION

Never tell the truth to people who are not worthy of it.

~ MARK TWAIN

Estheticians get pimples… on their butts, that is. And *that's* from sitting for hours on end (pun intended) doing what they absolutely and enthusiastically must do to realize their life's work, their dharma, their highest and holiest potential and zenithal beneficence; picking at your face. Now, if you *are* an esthetician, you know exactly what we're talking about and know you would rather get an "ass-cial" from your own BEF (Best Esthetician Forever) than have just anyone work on your face. And if you *have* an esthetician (or God forbid, you don't), then you probably don't know what the hell we're talking about right now or how this could possibly apply to you and your current beauty routine.

And this is *exactly* why you need this book. Because your esthetician doesn't tell you everything. Nope, they don't tell you about their pimpled posterior predicament, and some won't even share their own secret skincare strategies. Even more disheartening, they rarely tell you everything about your own skin.

Why not? Isn't this why you are spending your hard-earned cash in the first place? Not just for an hour of serenity and healing touch, but for their expertise? Their years of knowledge, training and down in the trenches experience so that you can figure out why you get a cyst on your chin every time you travel? Or how to banish brown blotches? Or why you woke up with lines around your lips when you are pretty damn sure they weren't there when you went to bed? So why the hell are they withholding?

Frankly, we don't have the balls. 98% of estheticians are women, and, like us, raised in a traditional female archetype to nurture, to please, to compliment, and to not say anything upsetting. So, what gave us the gumption after 30 combined years of working in the industry to say, "f*ck that shit" and lay it out? Here's the scoop.

Tanis' Story: When I was a wee lass, I spent my summers frolicking in the cool, lapping waters of the Colorado River where my family had a house in Needles, which just occurred to me was probably and appropriately named for that crazy jumping cholla (no, I did not say I got jumped by a chola – c'mon people, focus). I can still easily remember the smell of that water; an odd yet consistent blend of algae, earth, and an indescribable freshness never to be captured in any synthetic fragrance… not even Cool Water. The river bordered on chilly yet felt soothing on our parched, fried, blistered, and jacked-up skin. Ah, the Wonder Years… and now I wonder who had the sunscreen?

I inherited something from my father. Not just his fair hair and blue eyes, but also his dermatologist, who I met when I turned 18. Over 100 skin lesions whipped up, stitched up and biopsied later, my transition into the world of esthetics began. I came to understand that some stuff you inherit, and most of what you inherit that determines your health and beauty fate, are habits. And we can change habits, so pay attention.

Being a Nature Child and curious and creative as all hell, I studied science and earned a Bachelor's and a Master's Degree, naturally. These were the formative years when seeking facts and explaining the truth, often through collaboration (never competition) with other scientists, were deeply ingrained in me. I love biology and chemistry and the entire time I was researching, teaching, being Woodsy Owl (true story), doing lab work and carrying on in the science scene, I continued to get hacked up and pay for an excellent PPO plan so that I could maintain my rendezvous with my skin doc.

And then I met Valerie; my first esthetician. Before meeting her, I was a facial virgin and not only did she deflower me, she ignited a roaring blaze of obsession and OCD I had no idea was hiding under my hyperpigmented, whip-stitched, and prematurely aging skin. I was confounded by what my epidermis was doing and delighted to discover science had answers, and that there were remedies too.

I quit my corporate job and gave myself three months to blast through beauty school. I was going through a divorce and my future, particularly my financial future, was looking uncertain. For chrissakes, was I going through a midlife crisis? Probably. But for once (and many times thereafter), the scientist put her brain aside and decided with her heart that this was the right direction and damn the naysayers. By the time I went to take the State Board of Barbering and Cosmetology exam, I had a business plan, a three-treatment room spa in Eagle Rock, California, and a full-time job in the sciences, because a PPO is a good thing. Eighty-hour work weeks here I come.

So, why the compulsion to write a "tell all" skin book? Questions. I answered the same skincare questions over-and-over again. Also, because I noticed truthful answers were often surprising to whoever asked them, and so different from the inaccurate responses received from other sources.

After years of frustration, I sat down one morning with my cup of joe and wrote out 20 chapter titles for a book; the same ones you're about to read. I was going to be the one to give truthful answers to common and challenging skincare questions. Why?

1) I'm a scientist and base things on data–not feelings, someone else's false blog, or at-home experiments (well, at least not most of the time). I'm programmed to be factual and to tell the truth.

2) My esthetician, Valerie, was truthful with me when she told me my sunbathing, dehydration, and party habits were giving me melasma and pre-mature aging. She told me to "stop it!" To use her products, and I did. And it worked. And in the words of Mark Twain, "Never tell the truth to people who are not worthy of it." I guess Valerie thought I was worthy. And you are worthy, too.

Fourteen years later, I would not have had it any other way. So, it is with great exuberance and determination I tell you everything your esthetician *really* wanted to tell you…but didn't.

Neddy's Story: I entered the world amidst tall palm trees and cool oceanic breezes and grew up to the sounds of salsa music, Cuban food and Puerto Rican flags hanging from Dad's Chevy Citation mirror. I snacked on sweet plantains and watched my parents and their Caribbean friends, salsa dance until well after the witching hour, when there wasn't a dry shirt in the house. My parents infused the essence of their beloved islands into the heart and upbringing of their *mijita*.

And, no, my birthplace wasn't in the Greater Antilles. It was actually in Culver City, California, coined "Screenland" back then since it was one of the major movie-making centers of Los Angeles. When I was born, my family lived at The Culver Hotel, a historical landmark. The Culver built in the roaring '20s was charming and once owned by the legendary John Wayne. It still stands tall and formidable, like the Duke in the middle of Downtown.

In 1985, the year I was born, my folks were not living at The Culver because of its illustrious past and former prestigious residents. My story turns here, and the sparkle dulls. The hotel had hit a rough spot, so they converted it to low-income housing.

My Dad had just gotten hired as a city bus driver, and this was the first place he could afford. However, it was still a far cry from cold Chicago where my parents met; we counted our blessings. Our neglected hotel, although far from its glory days, was still a gem. We lived on the sixth floor, in the largest apartment on our level; which was a modest one bedroom. From birthday parties in the hotel hallways, to playing tag on the old yet magnificent marble staircase, to wondering when and if they would ever fix the elevator – it was a childhood home like no other.

Our large antique windows overlooked all that was famous and glamorous, but just out of reach. The rich views overlooking the former Desilu studios, Tara Mansion (from the film classic: Gone with the Wind), Sony Pictures, and MGM Studios complete with a giant Lion on top made my imagination wander. I grew up surrounded by movie magic and glamour. And from my first diaper-adorned toddle across a Hollywood Star of Fame I was completely enamored by it.

Being raised by a Cuban mother and grandmother, I grew up with an understanding of what it meant to be "Pretty in Pink," lady-like, and neat. Lessons in lip gloss application and cheek pinching preceded the necessity to tie my own shoes, first-things-first. Soon I was acting, modeling, and salsa dancing my way through childhood.

I knew what beat my heart was setting and my focus turned towards a career in Special Effects Makeup Artistry. I wanted to dive into the fantasy world I had gazed upon and imagined as a child from our high, sixth-floor window. I wanted to be a part of Hollywood filmmaking, and to create the most unimaginable images possible; from freaky aliens to slashed murder victims to glamorous princesses sequestered in lofty towers. I can still remember my mother screaming Spanish absurdities as she would catch me in the bathroom raiding her makeup, along with wads of toilet paper and water; papier-*mâchéing* my face and mimicking the techniques I saw on screen. It was no surprise to me, even though it was to everyone else when I skipped out on college and opted to go to makeup school in Hollywood instead.

Ay, Dios mio – once I began makeup school, often having practiced on myself, my skin became my frenemy, leading me to get my first professional facial with an esthetician named Nancy. I was twenty-one and by the time Nancy finished with me, not only did I have clear skin, I was also following a full skincare regimen. But the most important thing Nancy taught me was balance. I paid for her treatments and her invaluable advice every five weeks. Saving money from my paychecks (yup–said it, did it), to finance my skin therapy. After my skin cleared up, I saw her less, just as she planned, and then one day she moved away. I lost my secret weapon against breakouts, my skin mentor and confidant. Suddenly, I was a deer in headlights; albeit, with unblemished skin, but somewhat clueless.

I began my career in makeup with little to no knowledge about skincare except what I needed to do to get my skin in check. Eventually, after some growing pains, curiosity got the better of me and I joined the esthetics program at the same beauty school I had dropped out of during high school (yes, I was a beauty school dropout... oh, the humiliation). And yes, it happened to be right down the street from The Culver Hotel–FULL CIRCLE.

I love skincare because I adore how people feel after my treatments; I know that I am genuinely helping them solve not only their superficial skincare problems but what lays deep underneath, too; helping them strike a balance. These days, I'm devoting more time to curating master classes for estheticians and forging a great sisterhood with my mentor and dear friend, Tanis Rhines.

It's been an adventurous and star-lit journey this far, and yet I feel the ride's just getting started. Together, we have learned and shared many lessons; the most prominent "share" being the book you have in your hands. Why be so bold? Because I'm tired of making things "look pretty." Sure, it's fun and fantastical, but it's fake. It's time we step out of the screen and onto what's true and real. And the reality remains... the truth shall set you free!

PART I

WHY THE HELL AM I
BREAKING OUT?

"It is easy to display a wound, the proud scars of combat.
It is hard to show a pimple."

~ ANONYMOUS

It's a cold (but happy) day in hell when we have a client who proclaims that they do *not* break out. Skin is a living, functioning organ with glands and hairs and sebum and pus and blood. Almost all people experience congestion and then the predictable breakout, during some point in their life; and for many, throughout. There are different pimples for different people; everything from papules to pustules to secret hidden plugs. And for as many breakouts that can erupt, there are a million times more causes for them. But from garnering years of experience in the saddle stool of skincare, we think we may have squeezed it all and we certainly have researched and tried a myriad of remedies to help our physically and often emotionally afflicted clients.

Our Take: We can't count how many myths our clients are proclaiming as they lay on our treatment tables sharing their self-diagnosis of why that monster of a pimple is on their face! They are simply regurgitating what they read on a beauty blog or product ad as they turned to Google to answer the million-dollar question, "Why the hell am I breaking out?" Why is there so much misinformation out there about breakouts? Most advice we come across is a mosh of old wives' tales, marketing hype from slick ad campaigns mixed in with a dash of science and a sprinkle of data. Why aren't these omniscient advisors who claim they "know all, see all" actually telling you the truth?

Are they lazy? After all, it takes time and patience and a lot of thought to learn and understand everything about what is happening in the client's life that could cause pimple pandemonium. Everything from food intake to stress to nasty little habits to hormonal chaos needs to be considered, and that equals work.

Are they clueless? Many do not have formal schooling or training or licensing; they are simply repeating popular posts or even making stuff up as they go. Unfortunately, many estheticians are not skilled at administering remedies outside of the skincare lines with which they work.

Are they greedy? Many are slow to make suggestions that may cause them to lose a client or the money from the sale of a product. Most avoided, are the best FREE acne blasting remedies, items that can be picked up at the drugstore for $5, the recommendation to consult with a doctor, or *anything* that does not involve one of the fancy products on their shelf with a big profit margin and thin layer of dust.

Are they scared? Does your esthetician have the bollocks to tell you something that's not PC that makes them sweat and you blush so they can help you zap your zits? Look, no-one's out to hurt your feelings, but it's time for estheticians like us to truthfully tell you why you're breaking out and how you can get the clear and radiant skin you want.

We've decided to take that path, you know, the one a little tougher and less traveled, so we can offer you some pimple party crashers. We hope to scare the shit out of even your most formidable zit.

In these pages we're sharing our best advice and we hope for a clear future for our clients. Listen to what we're dishing and make your OWN decisions instead of just taking the word of a salesperson, blog post, YouTube clip, or dare we say, your own esthetician. Sit tight, relax, and get your dose of acne reality. It's time to binge read, so you can stop guessing and start clearing up.

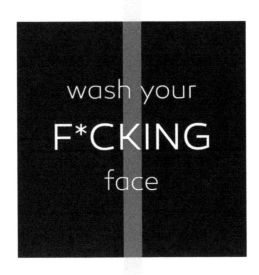

1

WASH YOUR F*CKING FACE

HONESTLY

This chapter is so important it was a contender for the title of this book. Why? Because it is *exactly* what your esthetician *really* wants to say to you, but doesn't. Probably the most asked question of estheticians is "How often should I get a facial?" The answer is twice per day, every day, if you don't wash your f*cking face! You know who you are—you're that person who is so incredibly lazy and cheap that you have talked yourself into believing you actually don't have to cleanse your skin regularly—meaning twice per day.

If you are one of these people, we're pretty sure your brain is already overflowing with excuses like "twice per day is too much because it strips your natural oils" or "my dermatologist told me that perfectly balanced skin does not need product." Or perhaps you are one of those who slip in a quick cleanse with that bar of green soap you've got hanging out in your shower. You know, the one you also wash your butt hole with that has enough wax and perfume to buff and shine half the cars in Ireland?

Or you think the shampoo you use in the shower that is loaded with harsh ingredients is "good enough" as it trickles over your face upon rinsing. To this behavior we respond… Get a Grip.

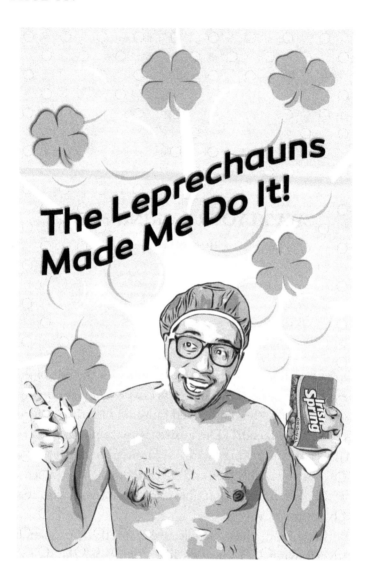

The Leprechauns Made Me Do It!

We have clients who do not wash their face and we can tell because it is oily, congested, smelly, gray, blotchy, and thick with dead waste (most people have 30 *extra* layers of dead cells on their face), blackheads, whiteheads, pustules, papules, small gerbils and an occasional wombat.

Here's some advice, while you're at it, just stop cleansing altogether. No soap for you. Just carry that post-workout, mid- menstruation, after sex stench around with you and see how that fares on your next job interview or Tinder date.

Your skin is being bombarded by muck and mire from the outside and oozing as a result from the inside. Here is a short list of items with perpetual visitation rights that are accumulating on your skin as you read this:

- **VOCs** (volatile organic compounds) are gaseous chemicals that emit from paint, glue and dry-cleaned clothes (to name a few sources). They can be skin irritants and carcinogenic.

- **SOx** (sulphur oxides) come from burning coal, extracting metals and refining petroleum. They are considered major air pollutants.

- **NOx** (nitrogen oxides) are found in car exhaust and cigarette smoke and are irritating and corrosive to the skin.

- **COx** (carbon oxides) increase when fossil fuels are burned and forests and coral reefs are destroyed. High levels can cause red and blistered skin.

- **Particulate Matter** is a major component of air pollution and leads to skin inflammation, premature aging and the breakdown of collagen… oh my!

- **Sweating** is good for the skin but when not cleansed off of the surface, the urea and ammonia in sweat can cause inflammation and irritation.

- **Sebum** helps protect the skin, but a buildup can cause acne and itchiness. Plus, it feeds microbes.

- **Bacteria, Yeast and Mold** are chomping away on that sebum and grimy feast laid out before them, a literal smorgasbord for them to party on and proliferate. Cleanse them away to ward off breakouts and rashes.

- **Microscopic Mites** creep about and inhabit your eyelashes, skin and nails. A zoo of these tiny insects can cause relentless itching and rashes.

- **Oils, Pigments, Petrochemical Derivatives, Preservatives, Herbicides, Pesticides** and godknowswhatelse arrive on the scene in your makeup and lotions and wreak havoc on skin.

But please, don't bother with washing your face. I'm sure all of your residents would rather you not. But for those of you convinced that washing the skin with an *appropriate* cleanser and lots of rinsing water is a good idea, we agree with you, salute you, and gladly offer tips.

What is cleansing? It is the removal of stuff you don't want. In the case of skin, it is the removal of dirt, oil and unwanted debris by using a soap. Will just water work? Not really. Remember your high school chemistry? 1) Like dissolves like and, 2) oil and water do not mix. Dirt, oil and most stuff chillaxing on our skin are oil-based. Since like dissolves like we will need something oil-based to grab onto the dirt. Oil and water do not mix, so trying to wash with just water won't work because the water will repel off the oil-based scum.

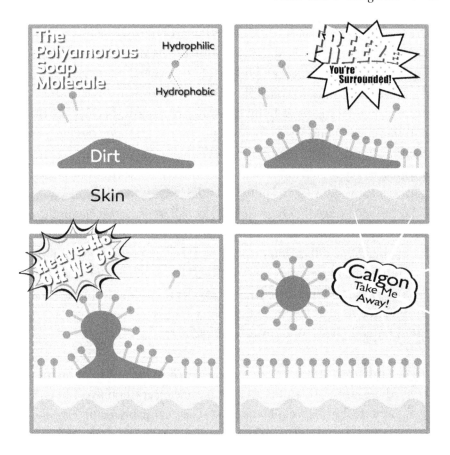

Enter the soap molecule (drum roll, please). The soap molecule is bipolar, not exactly like your college roommate, but basically the same. It has two different things happening at the same time. One end is water-like (we call that hydrophilic or "water loving") and will grab onto water molecules. The other end is oil-like (we call that hydrophobic or "water fearing") and will grab onto oily substances on your face; the dirt, oil, and debris. So, you mash up this soap with the face and the hydrophobic ends of the soap molecules hook up with all the junk on your face, swipe right. Then you splash water on your face and the hydrophilic ends of the soap molecules hook up with the water and it all washes away carrying with it the oil, dirt and debris, swipe right again. The polyamorous soap molecule is a double hook up! Hey, we didn't say it was exclusive.

What is soap versus a cleanser? First, both work as explained in our "chemistry of soap" lesson. In the esthetics industry, the definition of 'soap' is often misunderstood. Unless told otherwise, many estheticians may believe soap is a colorful, perfumed bar with surfactant for foaming. The fact is most body cleansing bar soaps, because of their harsh ingredients and waxy substances, are not good for the face, and sometimes not even for the body, especially for sud-sing your southern hemisphere. These substances can clog pores, and the perfumes, colors, and preservatives can act as potential allergens.

We're well aware that high quality, low allergen, facial cleansers are making a comeback in bar form, but we will still assume you are using Irish Spring if you tell us you use bar soap. For that reason, we will stick to the term "facial cleanser" or "cleanser" for products that are profile appropriate. A product labeled as a facial cleanser is made for your mug. You still need to give the ingredient list a once over to ensure you steer clear of harsh ingredients. Three to avoid are:

1) **Sodium Laurel/Sodium Laureth/Ammonium Sulfate,** these are surfactants that make cleansers bubbly. They can irritate skin, especially the eyes (yikes), cause breakouts especially around the mouth (lovely) and strip skin of its natural oils (*sigh*).

2) **Triclosan** this antimicrobial chemical may cause irritation and is a known endocrine disruptor (meaning it can mess with your thyroid and reproductive hormones). And besides, it may not work any better than good ol' soap and water!

3) **Colorants and Phthalate containing Fragrances** these are unnecessary and can be very irritating to skin. Phthalates are xenoestrogens and we tell you more later in this book, but for now, trust us when we say they are nasty. So, if you love your pretty pastel cleansers that smell delectable… best get over it.

What is the benefit of cleansing the skin? Cleansing removes oil and dead skin, making it easier for your products to penetrate deep down to the dermal layer where they do their best work. It removes pollutants and reduces the load of oxidative stress on the skin, which slows aging. It helps keep pores clear, allowing oil or sebum to flow onto the surface of your skin where it belongs; naturally protecting your skin from the harsh environment and microbial invaders. This decreases breakouts and keeps skin supple. Cleansing, especially when followed by a great moisturizing agent, keeps skin hydrated and at an optimum pH level. Hydrated skin is youthful skin. Plus, you won't stink and look like you have the starring role in "The Hills Have Eyes".

How to choose? This is where your professional esthetician comes in; the person who gets to see your face magnified 1000 times. She or he will lead you down the path of cleanser enlightenment.

Questions your esthetician should ask you:

- Do you have allergies or sensitivities?

- Will you use it to remove eye makeup?

- Do you need it to exfoliate?

- Do you want product with active ingredients to help calm, stimulate, brighten, tighten your skin?

- What is your budget?

- Are you using topical prescriptions?

- Do you give a damn about the health and vibrancy of your skin? Of course, you do, that is why you have an esthetician.

It is not possible for us to know every product out there, but a great esthetician will do a TON of homework before choosing the products they use and recommend. And out of the products they choose to use, they will be able to identify at least one cleanser, hopefully two, that will help you accomplish your skin care goals.

Tempted to hit your local drugstore or department store? Ok, but remember, most companies that sell through more mainstream methods (store fronts or online) spend a lot of money on packaging and marketing and not necessarily on the actual product in the container. How else are they going to get you to buy their product when it is sitting alongside hundreds of others? Yes, that supermodel advertising your favorite cleanser probably got paid more than the research, development, and ingredient cost of the stuff she claims to use and love. And she definitely got paid more than the formulation chemist (*sigh*) who crafted the stuff.

Here are a couple of tried-and-true cleansers that are wonderful for most skin types. The Botanique Bubbling Cleanser with a mild dose of AHA and BHA and calming botanicals gently swipe away debris while Tea Tree Oil helps to banish blemishes. For a dreamy cleansing experience, try the Citrus Cloud Cleanser with billowy mounds of foam infused with Grapefruit, and Green Tea for an antioxidant rich wash. Both cleansers by **NUÅGE9**®.

If you must hit the stores or shop online, be ready to decipher the ingredient list. Good luck with that. The words "organic" and "natural" do not mean that the products are devoid of petrochemical derivatives, mineral oil, animal parts and other interesting things you may not want on your face. General rules: avoid synthetic colors and fragrances (good luck with this one, too. This is how Big Beauty gets us to buy their shit because it is the cutest shade of pink and smells so deliciously good), stick to foamy and gritty if you are oily and tend to break out, and creamy is best for very dry skin. Beware of the oil-cleansing craze! Go read the chapter "Are You Old and White?". We have seen more hellacious breakouts from it than not.

When in doubt, find an esthetician that has a skin care philosophy similar to your own. Check out their "About" page on their website or give them a call. Do they use aggressive treatments, insist on a highly structured at-home regimen, favor organic products or make drugstore recommendations and with which one of these approaches are you most comfortable? And please ensure they are liberal with their advice. You wouldn't navigate the Amazon without a guide, would you? WOULD YOU?! And trust us… it's a jungle out there.

Tanis' & Neddy's Sidebar: Let's Keep It Clean

We are so passionate about cleansing that we try to do just a little to help with this issue and that is why we started the "Keep it Clean Campaign" that donates high quality facial cleansers to the Los Angeles Downtown Women's Center. We believe all people should have access to a cleanser and water for health, dignity and radiance. To find out more about this campaign for clean skin, go check out www.asktheestheticians.com.

WHAT YOUR ESTHETICIAN
REALLY WANTED TO TELL YOU

- Grow up and wash your f*cking face.

- If your face smells like Spring in the Land of Leprechauns, invest in a *real* cleanser… or go back to Ireland.

- Your skincare regimen begins with a quality cleanser. Avoid cheap fillers and harsh ingredients and pick one with active ingredients that are in line with accomplishing your skin care goals.

- Get a guide.

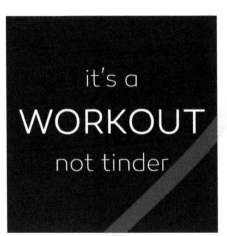

2

IT'S A WORKOUT – NOT TINDER

YOUR MAKEUP IS MESSING UP YOUR GOOD LOOKS

We've all seen it, a pretty young woman rushing into the gym to squeeze a workout into her jam-packed day. A runner dashing down the street to get in some cardio to keep those jeans zippable. We recommend exercise, sweating, and we passionately recommend profusely sweating while vigorously exercising. We want to commend these lovelies for making it happen in a hectic world. As we watch them and admire them for their commitment to a healthy lifestyle, we also see the telltale signs they are looking a bit *too* pretty to be pumped up. The skin that's just a little too even toned and contoured. The smoky eyes, the lined and painted mouth, the concealer over the bumps that are acne. Then we hang on the precipice, about to fall into the abyss of either empathy and compassion or pure unadulterated disdain.

You come to us because you have pimples. You have pimples because you wear makeup at the gym. You wear makeup at the gym because you are 1) lazy 2) insecure about your skin because you have pimples (because you wear makeup at the gym) and/or 3) you are more focused on the packs than the racks and use the gym as an opportunity to conduct a little swipe right, swipe left. Girl, we care and that is why workout time should be your time to decompress, get in shape, have fun, lose yourself in movement, attain goals, go introvert, listen to 80s hair bands, and lift. It is not the time to be rockin' the Kat Von D line and looking for Friday night's next big adventure.

This mash-up of makeup and workout may not seem like a big deal, but we are here to tell you it is, and why you need to immediately cease and desist. It's not that we aren't compassionate towards the young women who are embarrassed to leave the house without concealing the blemishes that make them feel insecure, frustrated, and less than their most magnificent selves. But you are going to have to break this cycle of wearing makeup when working out (or engaging in any sweaty activity), to get the clear skin you desire. Here's why…

Tanis' Take: I used to work as an environmental microbiologist. My job was to go to food production facilities, beverage companies, drug manufacturers, and places that made beauty products. I helped the facilities monitor the amount of microorganisms (bacteria, yeast and mold) in their factories and in their products… yes, I said IN the products. Some products, such as the drugs that are injected directly into our veins, must be sterile. That means absolutely NO microbes. Other products, such as many foodstuffs, must not contain certain types of microbes that cause food poisoning and potential death. One of these off-limit germs is *E. coli*. It's the bacteria that is found in feces and made McDonalds the first, but not last, fast-food restaurant to be awarded "free commercials" by the news stations in 1982.

And then… there are beauty products. The reigns of contamination are held a little more loosely in this sector. There are safeguards in place to prevent or inhibit the growth of microbes in products; using preservatives and low water activity means less of a chance that microbes will flourish. Low water activity means the more dry the product is, such as powdered eyeshadows, blush, and face powder, the less chance that microbes will survive and thrive in the product. Therefore, they will keep fresh for longer periods of time. When the water activity is high, such as in products like lotions, liquid foundation, shampoos, and conditioners, the greater chance that you're gonna get some unwelcome guests. When fingers are introduced into the mix you are adding a whole microscopic zoo to your facial products and really putting the preservative power of your product to the test. BTW, when tested in my microbiology class, the fingers of the students were more contaminated with microbes than their feet, even after walking barefoot to class.

Instead of sticking your fingers into
a jar, best to use a plastic or metal
spatula to dip in.

What's the point? Chances are there are some creepy critters in your cream that you are slathering all over your face. And we already know that the skin itself is covered with microbes. So, add a dash of makeup goo into the mix, bake at the gym for one hour, and those babies are gonna multiply faster than a newlywed Mormon couple. Next, stir in a fair amount of comedogenic (pore clogging) ingredients commonly found in makeup and you have created the ultimate pimple party.

Neddy's Take: I started my journey in the beauty business as a professional makeup artist (MUA) studying everything from beauty and corrective techniques to character and special effects makeup. The world of cosmetics has evolved immensely from my first days on set in the film and TV industry. With the introduction of YouTube, suddenly, makeup techniques were showcased and spotlighted. Next thing ya know, makeup was on fire like a Baked Alaska on a Caribbean cruise. Every self-proclaimed "Plain Jane" could now transform herself into her own supermodel, an artist with her own canvas. As a MUA, it was so exciting to see the surge of creativity! New MUA's and makeup influencers were popping up left and right; it was awesome to watch.

However, it's not necessary to see it "on parade" at the gym. Here's why: it really is detrimental to the condition of your lustrous skin! I remember when I was studying master makeup artistry in school; I was often my own model. Day in and day out, slathering, layering, powdering, and gluing products to my skin. The result? Moderate bouts with contact dermatitis, breakouts, itchy and irritated skin, and just friggin' dryness. I can't imagine doing a thirty to sixty-minute workout with a catwalk ready face. Many of the looks and techniques that we now use for everyday wear were not originally intended to be for *every* day. In the past, contouring would have been a little blush. Now, we are copying heavy makeup techniques that were only done in the entertainment industry during photo shoots, TV, film, and stage. The accentuated and defined features that would otherwise be washed out by harsh studio lighting could be achieved through the creation of shadow and light with our beloved cosmetics. These techniques kept images looking three dimensional. Now, everyone has access to these industrial strength contour kits, baking powders, tidal wave proof mascaras, and bullet proof concealers. Not to mention the extra 15 minutes tacked on to our regular makeup routines!

Yes, it's fun! I can admit that I, too, want to look as fabulous as RuPaul! But ladies, let's draw the line at the entrance to the gym. Give yourself, your skin, and your future flawless makeup-look a hand by washing off the Geisha face before SoulCycle®. First, it's dark in there. Second, don't even think for a hot second your skin can sweat through that industrial-strength mess. You'll be saving yourself from having to treat totally avoidable skin conditions. Embrace going bare while getting buff!

To help us steer clear of some nasty comedogenic ingredients commonly found in makeup, we made a list of "avoids."

Here are ten to watch out for:

1) **Acetylated Lanolin** this is oil from sheep, so not only is it non-vegan, it is highly comedogenic. It may also be listed as acetylated lanolin alcohol, athoxylated lanolin, PEG 16 lanolin, or the less common name of Solulan 16.

2) **Benzaldehyde is** a fragrance we can do without.

3) **Almond, Avocado and Wheat Germ Oil** try it on dry parts of the body, but avoid the face, chest and back where it may prove to be too rich.

4) **Shea Butter** ditto. We love it on elbows, knees, feet, shins… you get the picture.

5) **D&C Red** it will have a number. You should particularly avoid numbers 27 and 40 as they are rated as high on the clogging scale.

6) **Ethylhexyl Palmitate** also a fatty acid. Best go check your NARS® products, just sayin'.

7) **Isopropyl Palmitate** is a fatty acid found in many tinted moisturizers.

8) **Red Algae** it's trending and is found in some concealers but it is highly comedogenic and can be irritating to the skin.

9) **Lauric Acid** and/or **Coconut Oil** we know you know we are coconut heads, but we don't want to be broken out coconut heads. Eat coconut oil, put it on your body, but you better avoid makeup with these two topical, tropical storm ingredients.

10) **Isopropyl Myristate** is a conditioning agent that may leave your skin in bad condition!

So, here's what you do Dancing Queens: throw a couple of things in your gym bag and save face.

1) Carry a very gentle, use-all-over-your-face foaming cleanser, like **Kiss My Face® Hand Soap**. Hold on the judgment, sister. We know it's called hand and not face soap, but Tanis has been using this to obliterate her Tammy Faye Bakker mascara jobs since a fellow forest ranger introduced her to it in 1990. And yes, you can emulate Ms. Bakker and still simultaneously be a bang-up ranger 'because that's how badass babes roll.' Just remember to wash that shit off *before* you get in the Woodsy Owl costume you are wearing to the campfire program or you'll be looking like Marilyn Manson gone bobbing for apples.

Anyway, they recently changed the name from Face Soap to Hand Soap, but everything else stayed the same, including its mascara melting abilities. You can usually find this product in health food stores, so it's our go-to if we forget our typical make-up remover when we are traveling. Get the unscented.

2) Give **Eminence® Stone Crop Cleanser** a spin; super gentle and smells like a fresh field of, well, stone crop.

3) A go around with a cleanser ain't cutting the eye job? Grab a cotton ball and a Q-tip with one of these products and swoosh goes the eyeliner. Try Eminence® Rice Milk 3-in-1 Cleansing Water (water based) or **Fitglow® Makeup Cleansing Oil** (oil based). We do NOT know how we got it all off before we discovered these makeup melters.

4) Finish the job with **Pharmaskincare® Botanica Vit Complex Exfoliant** to scrub off any last trace of foundation while simultaneously giving your skin a little boost of salicylic acid to kill off any hangoners.

You are now ready to dump a deluge straight outta yo' face. Congratulations! You've done such a world-class job of decontaminating your dermis you only need a thorough rinsing and maybe a swipe with a toner at the *end* of your workout. Still feeling lazy or need to meet up with Swipe Right post-gym? Skip the eye makeup removal, but do NOT skip sud-sing your skin. Mr. Right will thank you. Hoot!

WHAT YOUR ESTHETICIAN
REALLY WANTED TO TELL YOU

- The gym is not a supermodel runway or pick-up joint. Save the beauty routine for a less sweaty situation.

- Thoroughly wash your face *before* beginning your exercise routine.

- Use plastic or metal spatulas to dip creams out of jars; your fingers are highly contaminated with bacteria, yeast and mold.

- Avoid comedogenic ingredients in your makeup.

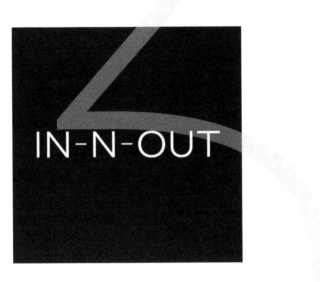

3

IN-N-OUT

WHAT GOES IN IS GONNA COME OUT... OF YOUR FACE

"OMG! Don't hate me because I know you see that grease from my
2am run to Tommy's when I got a little tipsy with my girls. I just know
there's chili cheese fries oozing out of my pores! I woke up in a puddle,
a full oil boil; ground cow, cheddar, fried spuds and all. Please make
it stop and I swear I will NEVER eat those perilous potatoes again!"

~ FOOD SIN CONFESSION #1,267

How many times have you heard that your diet affects your skin? We
can remember the rules oh so clearly: "No Sweets, No Grease, No
Dairy!" Yet it's almost daily we are questioned by our clients if it's *really*
true? And if so, why can some people eat whatever they want and never
see a pimple, compared to others who face the uphill battle of life with
acne? But also, is it just about pimples? Does eating pizza really create
a pizza face? Before your next fast food run, think twice. We're diving
"face first" into this topic and clearing the slate, and hopefully your
face, once and for all!

As easy as it would be to just say, "yes, junk food is to blame for your
acne, wrinkles and aging, so STOP NOW!" We would be lying, even

if it was a small white lie for your own good. We're not your Mama, so we'll spare you the scolding. And to our frustration, this is still very much up for debate in the world of dermatology. Many Dermatologists dismissed such ideas as mere myths. But after a combined skin practice of over 25 years, we say hold the presses we have seen years of evidence, including on our own skin, that show what goes in, eventually seems to come back out.

This chapter is not about the hormone imbalances and glucose sensitivities caused by a body that is biochemically imbalanced because of obesity, epigenetic factors, or other major challenges. For more info on that, read "Your Weight is Over." It is also not about drug indulgences such as cocktails, coke-tales, herbal refreshments or any scripts that your doctor has prescribed (or a trip down to Mexico has afforded you).

This chapter is about the food we eat: the good, the bad, the delicious, the indulgent, the 2am Taco Bell, the Sunday eggs benedict avec mimosas, and your mama's pot roast dinner. It's about the countless food decisions we make every day of our lives. This gets complicated, it gets emotional, and it gets real. Food affects your skin organ just like it affects all the other organs and systems in your body. Cool thing and crappy thing about it affecting your skin is that "it shows."

This can be a useful way to monitor when something is really nutritious and supports detoxification and health. It also means when you are eating like a junk-food-junkie and it's leading to inflammation, mucus production, congestion and wrinkles... your friends are going to be in-the-know. Are you ready to hear the truth your esthetician may have been too afraid to even tell themselves? Of course, you are. That's why we're here. Let's begin.

Fact or Fallacy? NO SWEETS

Let's define sweets. This might be painful because it's more than just what's in the candy aisle. It includes a couple of aisles to the left, a few more to the right, a good portion in the freezer and not to mention the refrigerator cases at the grocers. Damn. But wait, there's more. Yes, the liquor section, where Tanis has been known to disappear for hours at a time, perusing the latest release of Beaujolais. Does this also include fruit? Yes, but to a lesser extent based on the fiber and sugar load of the particular fruit, but it definitely includes juice. Before you go getting hangry with us, here's the scoop.

Here's a brief lesson about carbs
and the many faces of sugar.

Let's break it down, literally. Carbohydrates are long chains of sugars. They include combinations of the simple sugars: glucose, fructose, and galactose. They can come in pairs or long chains, but when your body breaks them down, the end result is sugar. Sugar stimulates the insulin response that is amazing, necessary, and complicated. The types of sugar, the amount of fiber, your genetics, among other things, affect your personal insulin response. It's been a while since Tanis taught biochemistry, so we're keeping it simple. Let's focus on what it means when we are overdoing it with sugar and experiencing frequent insulin responses. In other words, when you are eating too many damn carbs and it's jacking up your face.

Too much sugar equals inflammation, which creates oxidative stress, feeds cancer cells, increases hormone secretions, and erupts skin. Our noshes can damage DNA and collagen, creating fine lines, wrinkles and an aged appearance. Plus, according to a 2014 study in *The Journal of Drugs in Dermatology*[3], refined carbs are the primary culprit in the rise of adult acne cases.

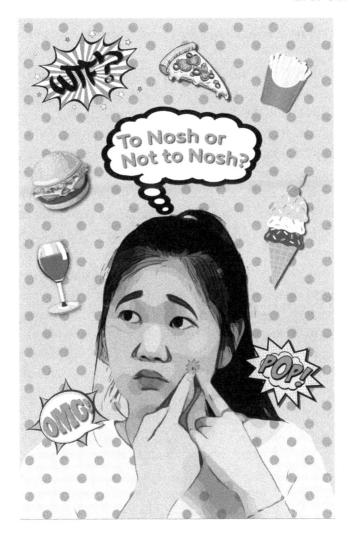

A recent study suggesting a link between diet and acne has "created a tidal wave in the dermatology community," says Loren Cordain, a professor of health and exercise science at Colorado State University in Fort Collins. "If you look at the medical textbooks on dermatology, specifically the medical texts on acne, it's spelled out loud and clear that diet has NO effect on acne," he says. We say - say wha??? Clearly the people who wrote the texts on dermatology never owned a skin care clinic or had a brain.

When Tanis was in college, she was a vegetarian. Like many, her diet consisted of mainly carbs: pasta, crackers, breads, pita bread, bagels,

English muffins, etc. Acne quickly ensued. Several years and cases of benzoyl peroxide later, she switched to raw veganism, eliminating all bread substances from her diet and poof, within two weeks, no more acne. Upon speaking with other clear skinned raw vegans, all reported the same. Duh. And diet has no effect on acne? Really?

Cordain and colleagues concluded that consumption of candy bars, potato chips, cookies, doughnuts, cakes, soda, pizza, white breads, and other processed sugary and starchy foods common to Western cultures may indeed have an effect! The researchers arrived at their findings after studying 1,200 Kitavan Islanders of Papua New Guinea and 115 Ache hunter-gatherers of Paraguay. "We didn't find a single case of acne," Cordain says[4].

Is a western diet to blame? In the USA, acne afflicts about 80 to 95 percent of teens and even middle-aged adults. In search of an explanation, the researchers examined the diets of the two primitive cultures. The Kitavan Islanders ate mostly fish, fruit, tubers and almost no processed foods, while the Ache hunter-gatherers consumed primarily vegetables, peanuts, rice, some wild game and only a small amount of pasta, bread and sugar.

Cordain strongly believes their diet is the reason they had no acne. Specifically, they rarely ate refined carbohydrates like breads and sweets that have a "high glycemic load" meaning they cause blood sugar levels to surge.

A steady diet of such foods can trigger a "hormonal cascade" that leads to acne, according to Cordain's theory. High blood sugar levels cause the pancreas to pump out more insulin, which triggers the release of male hormones and growth factors. In the end, Cordain says, more oil is produced and more skin cells slough off, clogging pores.

While it's possible that good genes help these populations have clear skin, he says, other groups of Pacific Islanders and South American Indians who move to areas where Western diets are common develop acne. Previous observations have indicated the same thing happened when Eskimos started eating Western foods.

Carbs to Enjoy: here is a list of some lower glycemic carbohydrates we personally like to eat.

- Berries. Cherries. Grapefruit. Limes. Lemons.

- Bulgur wheat. Yes, it has gluten, but who gives a shit. If you don't have Celiac disease or wheat sensitivity, go for it.

- Pasta. Especially ones made from shiratake (flour from the konjac plant) or tofu. BTW, shiratake noodles are carb and CALORIE free! And if you can find it, Bella Bondonza™ pasta made from organic green beans and water (no joke).

- Ancient grains. Quinoa, amaranth, buckwheat and brown rice.

- Steel-cut oats. Try them savory!

- Peas. Mmmmmm... Pea salad...

Carbs to Avoid: look above. If it's not on that list, think twice before putting it in your mouth. Is that a berry you're holding? No? PUT IT DOWN. Wine Time? Change that to a Kettle One® straight up with a twist. Yes, please. NO SUGAR, FACT!

Fact or Fallacy? NO GREASE

Food's effect on the skin does not necessarily mean that what goes in will literally squirt right back out. Like our Food Sin Confession, we often hear our clients as they swear their midnight Chicken & Waffles attack came a-pouring out of their pores. Even though it seems like this may sometimes be the case, several studies show that downing greasy foods does NOT create breakouts (but getting that grease ON your face can make an oily complexion worse, clogging pores and leading to zits, so just don't face plant your pepperoni pizza).

For all of those times when your mama screamed at you about how eating all that greasy, fried, delectable, mouth-watering, comforting (oh we digress) food was to blame for that monster on your mug, or your second third eye, she was mainly watching out for your diet, silently hoping it would clear your skin. Blame the obvious, Parenting Handbook #1. But as teenagers, our sebaceous glands rev up due to hormones producing extra oil, creating shiny noses and foreheads, clogged pores and eventually zits. It's the comedones, not the cheese-on-a-stick, that lead to the breakout. Even as adults, we embrace the fallacy, ignoring the fact that acne has more to do with hormones, sugar and genetics than it does grease. Some foods WILL alter your hormones (Read No Sweets No Dairy) but oil is not a primary culprit.

So, eat away and savor your deep-fried wontons, bacon wrapped everything, country fried steak... breakout free. And be sure to enjoy your high cholesterol, impotence, strokes, angina and early onset death. Bon appétit! NO GREASE... FALLACY!

Fact or Fallacy? NO DAIRY

Ditch the dairy. Not only does it create phlegm, inflammation, and speed up aging, it's also associated with an increased risk of acne. And unfortunately, we are not just talking about milk. We're talking about walking away from the cheese table at the wine tasting. Yeah, we mean the baked brie.

We're suggesting skipping Yogurtland® and FroYo® because just when we thought we had a "healthy" dessert, it's messin'. We're thinking your famous Super Bowl 7 Layer Dip is now 5 layers. We're talking about a Bailey's Irish with no cream. Hot chocolate with no milk. Toast with no butter. DRY cereal. A study that followed a group of teenagers for three years found those that who drank more than two servings of milk per day were 20% more likely to suffer from acne than those who drank less than one serving per week[5]. An Italian study conducted on young adults concluded there is a 78% higher risk of acne for those drinking more than three servings per week[6].

Oh, but wait! Opposite Land Alert... all of the dairy studies cited indicate that FAT FREE milk exacerbated skin conditions MORE than the full/part-fat milk[7]. Things that make you go "hmmmm."

Hey, even when Nestles® admits milk causes acne, can you still say "N-E-S-T-L-E-S makes the very best"?

This never happened to Tanis' peaches and cream (pun intended) cheeked Fräulein living on her family's German farm. But hey, they were drinking raw straight from a warm titty. So what happens between the nipple and the carton? Go read our take on raw milk. But pasteurized or not, research in the past two decades has explained the role hormones play in acne; especially insulin and insulin-like growth factor 1 (IGF-1). Higher hormone levels usually mean higher acne levels. The link to dairy? Studies show that milk and other dairy products increase IGF-1 levels. One study in older adults showed that three servings of milk per day for 12 weeks increased IGF-1 levels by 10%[8].

Dairy cows have naturally occurring higher levels of hormones, like progesterone and IGF-1 (no surprise) which are making them lactate in the first place. In our modern world, cows are also spiked with additional hormones such as recombinant bovine growth hormone (rBGH) or recombinant bovine somatotropin (rBST) which increases the levels of IGF-1, and makes them produce even more milk.

Therefore, more milk (especially skim) from cows treated with more hormones probably means a higher IGF-1 level for you. This leads to acne breakouts and to possibly higher levels of prostate, breast, and other cancers. While there may be a link between IGF-1 blood levels and cancer, the exact nature of this link remains unclear. There are many research scientists who have devoted their life's work to studying the effects of this interesting hormone, so we encourage you to do your own research and keep up to date as new data arrives on the scene. Meanwhile, what we do know is it can lead to increased levels of inflammation, aging and gives men higher chances of colorectal cancer; in addition to acne[9]. Milk… it does a body "good." NOT.

Raw Dairy: If you love milk, research raw! Listen, for those of you who adore dairy, there may be a silver lining (to be explored at your discretion). Dairy does have a bad rap when it comes to acne and skin inflammation. However, there have been multiple reports and studies that conclude that the benefits of raw milk are plentiful. There are even those who consume raw milk to ease skin conditions such as psoriasis, eczema, and acne. How can this be?

First thing to note is that raw milk has *not* been pasteurized, which is the process of heating the product to kill harmful bacteria. This is a controversial topic, as the FDA and CDC are against unpasteurized dairy products. But please ponder that the pasteurization process kills beneficial bacteria in conjunction with denaturing important enzymes and proteins. We encourage you to find a reputable raw dairy distributor and ensure that the animals are strictly grass-fed and raised in humane conditions.

Here are some raw milk benefits to consider: It contains large amounts of Omega-3 fats and healthy saturated fats, which support skin hydration. This would explain the growing beauty trend of goat's milk soap bars and moisturizers hitting the U.S. market. Probiotics in raw milk can kill off or balance bad bacteria in your gut, significantly improving the health of your skin. Research has shown that inflammation and unbalanced gut flora do in fact, play a part in skin conditions such as acne, eczema and rosacea.

This is obviously not suitable for those that have dairy and/or milk intolerances. We should also note that ingested raw milk is not best for infants, young children, the elderly, pregnant women, and people with weakened immune systems. And even though raw is not recommended for babies and toddlers, we have an interesting story we want to share. Growing up in the (then) dairy community of Cerritos, California, a newborn Tanis refused to breastfeed, despised formula and poo-pooed cow's milk. This bright-eyed bundle of joy was soon becoming a "shrinking Thumbelina" as baby Tanis increasingly lost weight.

The magic trick to getting this persnickety tot back on track? A local farm happened to have some raw goat's milk that she gratefully guzzled down, which could explain why you don't stand between her and the goat cheese log at a party. Moral of the story: raw milk is different from pasteurized. Goat milk is different from cow's milk. Almond, coconut, soy and cashew milk are not milk at all and offer amazing tasting lactose-free vegan options. There's a big "milk" universe out there, people, go drink it!

Do take extra care if choosing to consume raw dairy. But we would say it's worth the research for any acne-prone dairy lovers! Go rogue! Are you cautionary? Then jump on the goat bandwagon! No, we don't mean doing yoga with one like Khloé Kardashian. We mean adding some product au lait to your everyday skincare regimen.

This milk is loaded with lactic acid, an excellent exfoliator that pumps up the moisture content of skin while reducing sallowness and spots. Check out **Beekman 1802**® as their nanny goat juice infused mercantile is extensive, ranging from beauty to home goods to cheese to shaving creams. Yup, everything dope that's goat can be found on their page at www.beekman1802.com.We recommend starting with the Pure Goat Milk Essentials Box Set that even includes a shampoo bar and cuticle cream. See if this farm-to-face beauty secret works wonders for you! Bleeeaaaat. NO DAIRY... YOU DECIDE.

Tanis' & Neddy's Sidebar: In-N-Out

Tanis' Take: When I first started in esthetics, I was the scientific version of Doubting Thomas. "Food cannot possibly affect the condition of the skin," I was known to pontificate. I was very fond of soap boxing, albeit with my dehydrated, hyperpigmented, pimply little face. After all, "food is broken down to its primary components in the digestive tract, cleaned and purified by the liver and kidneys and waste is excreted while the nutrients are used to build, nourish and reconstruct." And yes, that basic explanation is factual. At that time, I did not understand the nuances and the sometimes tremendous impact food has on our skin, body, and even mental states (Google: Raw Veganism and Schizophrenia). After years of practicing esthetics, raw veganism, exercise, massage, yoga, meditation and sauna, I can confidently state, "What the hell was I thinking?" Food absolutely has a dramatic effect on the overall vibrance, energy levels and aging process of the body. I have seen clients go from high carb diets as a vegetarian and shift to a raw vegan diet and watch their skin immediately clear. I have watched clients give up dairy, refined sugars and even heavy greasy meat and see their skin heal, shine and glow. As a good scientist, I cannot ignore 14 years of direct experiential research. Hippocrates, you had this one right.

Neddy's Take: Growing up Latina, sometimes the science and nuances of the relationship between food and skin went unnoticed. In fact, I didn't really know much about the physiology of the skin at all (until I enrolled in beauty school), much less what triggered its fluctuating conditions. But I do remember, oh so fondly, when an annoying bugger would show up on my face. The answer? To me, some soap, a needle, peroxide, and an overnight blob of toothpaste! I had chronic dry flakey skin and a Rudolph nose! Could my diet have something to do with this? Well, let me put it this way, I was a soda drinking, chip chomping, carb-o-holic! Were these devilish delights seeping out of my pores? Of course not! But was it chipping away at the overall condition of my skin? Absolutely. So I put my big girl chonies on and changed up my diet, trading my soda for good ol' H_2O and my chips for cucumber slices. My skin halted on the highway to hell and made a U-turn auto-cruising into a JLO glow. Although it may feel like death changing your diet, it's well worth it... because flipping off the grim reaper with a clear face is so much more fun! Clean up your habits and you'll clear up your skin.

WHAT YOUR ESTHETICIAN
REALLY WANTED TO TELL YOU

- Sometimes we can't help you until you want to help yourself. Are you ready to change the way you eat in order to slow aging, increase energy and stamina, and enjoy vibrant, clear skin? No? Then we can't help you either. If yes, put down the Ding Dong and contact Tanis on Facebook at Ask the Estheticians. She provides nutritional skin counseling to clients; especially the raw vegan curious.

- Let food be thy medicine, and medicine be thy food. Okay, that was Hippocrates, but your esthetician wants to say it too.

- For clear skin: if you want 'the in' but are afraid of 'the out', eat that burger "protein style" and pass on the bun, maybe the cheese; split the fries with a friend and just say no to the sugary shake. Your skin (and friend) will thank you.

- Don't lie to us. We can see in your pores what you had for lunch (wink-wink).

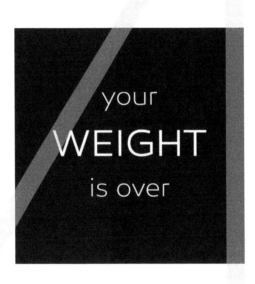

your
WEIGHT
is over

4

YOUR WEIGHT IS OVER

YOUR PUDGE IS MAKING YOU PIMPLY

A person's weight is a very personal subject, particularly if addressed on the facial treatment table. This is supposed to be a relaxing experience for the client, a "Calgon Take Me Away" moment when the recipient gets a break from reality and takes a mini personal time out. But when we see jawline and neck breakouts with obesity and increased facial hair growth, we really want to tell them why they are probably breaking out. But we don't. Why is being overweight so off limits as a topic? After all, hygiene is also a personal topic but discussed openly and passionately during the facial.

"Do you wash your face, how often, with what product?" When we see clients with a new crop up of breakouts around the mouth, even questions like "do you have a new boyfriend? Because that certainly looks like some make-out break-out to me!" That's acceptable, but weight… hmmm. Well, statistically, parents would rather talk about sex, drugs, and rock 'n roll with their kids than their eating habits.

According to a "Raising Fit Kids" survey conducted by the WebMD/ Stanford University FIT program, 22% of parents are uncomfortable talking about the risks and consequences of being overweight[1]. Surprisingly, other prickly parent-child topics that make moms and dads wince don't rank nearly as high. For parents of teens, the topic of sex ranked second place at 12%, smoking and drugs third at 6%, and alcohol placed fifth on the list at 5%. So, who's supposed to talk to your kids about being overweight? It's their doctors' job, 19% of parents say. Yet only 1% of parents think it's primarily a doctor's job to talk to their kids about sex, drugs, or alcohol. Talk to my kids, don't talk to my kids. But what we want to know is who the hell is talking with YOU?

Similar to parents with their children, estheticians would rather NOT talk with their clients about their extra weight. Actually, we really don't give a damn about your weight and we hope you return the favor; we both own a mirror and a scale. But this is a chapter in our book because when our clients ask us what is causing their breakouts and after extensive questioning and thorough consideration, we have come to the almost certain conclusion that it is their diet, it is time we speak the truth. We are telling it like it is with the chance that our candidness will help you not only attain your skin goals but your optimum health (which is oh so much more important).

Being overweight, particularly for females, can create hormonal hell. The excess weight combined with avoiding exercise can affect hormone levels, which can, in turn, impact the skin and overall health. Our Standard American Diet (SAD) is chock full of the "S" word, sugar. Bread, tortillas, pasta, cereal (even your steel-cut oats), granola bars, most protein bars and rice are all carbohydrates that trigger an insulin response and break down into sugar in our bodies. Sneaky. And then there is the obvious: cookies, ice cream, chocolate, and cake, which contain simple sugars the most detrimental to our health. Even our coffee can be chock full of it. Yes, our half-decaf-caramel-chocolate latte with whipped cream spikes blood glucose, that can lead to breakouts, insulin resistance, and eventually conditions such as Type II Diabetes and other life-threatening health conditions.

Carbohydrate heavy diets and inflammatory foods can cause insulin to surge, messing with the delicate balance between estrogen and testosterone. If you're a Sugar Queen, birth control pills may not even work to address breakouts. In 2012, they released the results of a study that analyzed the relationship between weight gain and acne in over 3,500 teens aged 18 or 19 who lived in Norway. Not surprisingly, the epidemiologists concluded that with a higher weight, the frequency of acne increased, too[2]. So, what is the actual relationship between excess weight and breakouts?

Let's consider what makes a zit. Your skin is constantly shedding. As it grows, the cells push outward and then eventually fall off; especially when assisted with a good cleanse and exfoliation. Inside a pore, however, we experience "opposite land" and the cells that line the inside of the pore move in and down instead of up and out. These flakes of dead skin will accumulate on the bottom of the pore and when everything is working just dandy, will be flushed out when the pore releases sebaceous oils; the oil carries the dead skin away and everybody lives happily ever after. But, when testosterone levels are high, the pores make more oil. This large volume of oil can puddle in the bottom of the pore, pulling it down, making the neck of the pore narrower. The dead cells that would normally get a ride out in a stream of sebum accumulate at the bottom of the pore.

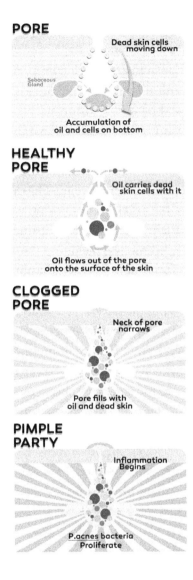

PORE

Dead skin cells moving down

Sebaceous Gland

Accumulation of oil and cells on bottom

HEALTHY PORE

Oil carries dead skin cells with it

Oil flows out of the pore onto the surface of the skin

CLOGGED PORE

Neck of pore narrows

Pore fills with oil and dead skin

PIMPLE PARTY

Inflammation Begins

P.acnes bacteria Proliferate

As the opening of the pore gets even more narrow, the skin grows over the top of the opening and *voilà*, you've got yourself a whitehead. The oil solidifies and forms a plug.

If the top of the plug is exposed to oxygen, the grease will oxidize and turn black and then you've got yourself a blackhead. And if you're really lucky and *P. acnes* bacteria get stuck in there and proliferate your body's immune system kicks in sending inflammatory compounds to the site, you're gonna end up with a big juicy pustule or an underground cyst. Yikes! I guess the next question would be "then what causes excess testosterone?" Glad you asked. Sugar.

When we eat sugar, insulin carries glucose all over the body. If there is too much sugar (think all-you-can-eat breadsticks alongside your spaghetti dinner followed by a little tiramisu, oh, and a glass of wine) most cells throughout your body can shut down their glucose receptors so they aren't flooded with sugar that needs to be metabolized creating dangerous free radicals. The 'key' words are "most cells." Guess which organ cannot block the entry of extra sugar? The ovaries. When all your other tissues are kickin' the crack, your poor little ovaries get drowned in cane, which makes them freak out. The insulin triggers cells in the ovaries to over-produce hormones, including testosterone. Hello acne, ruddy skin, unwanted facial hair, and weight gain. And even though breakouts and an increase on the scale occur, it's really the presence of sugar that's creating the pimple party.

Some of the worst acne we see is in females with a condition known as polycystic ovarian syndrome (PCOS) or Stein-Leventhal syndrome. PCOS is a disorder in women characterized by an elevated level of male hormones (androgens) and infrequent or absent ovulation (anovulation). This condition occurs when ovaries are overstimulated, usually by an influx of sugar from the bloodstream. The ovaries make more than the usual amount of both estrogen and testosterone, and the testosterone keeps oil glands overactive all the time. This can cause a cessation in menstruation or irregular periods so the breakouts do not even cycle with the period, they just persist. The excess testosterone production may also cause excess facial hair growth.

The simplest way to correct PCOS is to correct insulin sensitivity. This can be done with drugs, or it can be done naturally with an adjusted diet. Lowering the amount of sugar in the bloodstream, even slightly, can help the ovaries stop making excessive amounts of testosterone. Normal periods may be restored, and acne and hair growth stopped.

Just losing 2-3% of total body mass (4-5 pounds in most women) through calorie reduction usually is enough to restore hormonal balance. Menstrual cycles regulate and fertility returns about the same time acne disappears. This approach only works if women eat less and consume less sugar. Adding in exercise without the weight loss does not have the same effect. Period. But you can reduce sugar intake and lose a little weight to shake off breakouts for good.

Tanis' Take: This chapter is really not about your skin, it's about your health and possibly your survival. My 55-year-old aunt suddenly died from a weight related heart attack. I miss her terribly. I want you to thrive and experience your life to the fullest (and yes, look great doing it). This is a personal matter and I care about you, personally, and that is why I want to share this information. I want you to be healthy and set the example for your children, students, nieces and nephews to end the obesity epidemic in this country. They are watching what you eat and eating what you prepare. Talk to them about food. Be a rebel against the Standard American Diet, slash sugar, and reap the benefits. For optimal health and vibrancy, try a plant-based diet, or as close to it as you dare, by replacing processed carbs, meat, and dairy with fresh fruits, legumes, and raw or blanched vegetables. Contact your doctor or consult with a nutritionist to get started and then just do it. And if you are raw vegan curious, contact me. I am here to help. I support you. Don't make me terribly miss you.

Neddy's Take: Whoa, that's A LOT to take in and much easier *said* than *done*. However, it is not impossible. Take it from a Caribbean Latina, who loves her fair share of meat, plantains and immense amount of carbs (processed or not). Food has been a part of the integral family dynamic for many cultures around the world and being able to share in a home cooked meal with relatives is a form of love. "Breaking bread in fellowship" is literally that; a way to build intimate relationships. Even in our current culture, how many business deals, hot dates, birthdays and numerous other social gatherings take place around food or in a restaurant?

Not to mention, food can be a source of comfort for many. I mean, the term "comfort food" is a common term because it is often tied to our emotions. It's our escape from stress, sadness, or anxiety (I know, I've been known to dive into some junk food to ease a broken heart).

But it's not all negative, it goes both ways. We use food to celebrate victories, too (cake anyone?)! But let's get a reality check. Food habits don't just happen to you, they're a choice. The reason I say it's not impossible, is because after all, YOU are in the driver's seat. It takes much dedication, discipline, and self-forgiveness, but you don't have to be a victim of your food flaws. It's best to start with a visit to your doctor, then little by little, while being mindful of your habits, be willing to change the unhealthy ones. While you are at it, look at the other parts of your life that may need adjusting. After all, we often eat to fill a void within ourselves that has nothing to do with food. Remember that active bodies and positive minds have less stress and worry. By exercising your passions (do you have a hobby you love?), and maintaining an overall balanced lifestyle, you'll find that your inclination to binge eat will decrease. Have I given up my meat, plantains, and carbs? No. But I have changed the frequency of when I partake in those indulgences. I swap out my junky cravings for healthy alternatives. Is it easy? Not always. But is it worth it? Always.

WHAT YOUR ESTHETICIAN **REALLY** WANTED TO TELL YOU

- WE CARE about your health and your skin. See a doctor if you are overweight. You deserve a healthy, beautiful body and if we think you deserve it, you should, too. Consult a health professional or nutritionist to begin your journey.

- Extra sugar triggers extra estrogen and testosterone and can lead to hormonal imbalances creating breakouts. If you are overweight and breaking out, your time and money are best spent on getting fit first, your skin will follow.

- In severe cases, extra weight leads to Type II Diabetes and/or PCOS and with that, acne, unwanted facial hair growth and infertility.

- Make this simple, choose health. We are here to help. Besides a visit with your doc, other resources are available to aid you in your journey. We suggest finding a health coach in your area that focuses on the body-mind, soul connection. So much inspiration is just a click away!

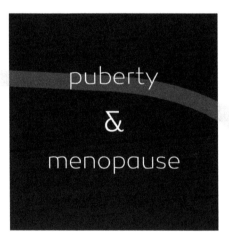

puberty

&

menopause

5
_____

PUBERTY & MENOPAUSE

S.O.S – SAME OL' SITUATION

Sorry ladies, if you thought you only had to ride on the hormonal highway to hell once in your life, you better swallow a reality pill because you ain't seen nothing yet. Yeah, you were full of teenage angst, whipsawed by confusion, and wanted to "kill" your mother and possibly yourself, but at least the first time you rode this roller coaster you were young and full of energy, slept through the night, late into Saturday morning, with a few midweek naps thrown in for good measure, had firm skin and your boobs were still in your northern hemisphere. We hope and pray that your exit out of fertility-land is graceful, easy and short.

Unfortunately, with most women working two to three full-time jobs (one or two outside the home and one in the home) either with or without a partner around, our fried out adrenal glands and frazzled out nerves set us up for an early onset, long and completely messed up menopausal experience. We work with thousands of clients who are suffering through this transition, some of whom never quite exit out of (we have family members still having hot flashes in their 70s)!

If menopause is degrading your quality of life to the point where you cannot function, have chronic insomnia, can't cut through the brain fog, are experiencing a radical negative impact on your job and/

or relationships or you just feel hopeless, we implore you to talk to a doctor who is WELL VERSED in bio-identical hormone replacement therapy to see if it can help you through the change. We care and want women to be empowered, creative, vibrant, strong and healthy (both mentally and physically) into their hundreds! But meanwhile, let's talk about your skin and what happened when you entered the fertile zone and why it may start all over again upon your exit.

Why does our skin go berserko when we go through hormonal changes? Doesn't it feel like those breakouts are a signal to the outside world to stay away? They're like a neon sign flashing that we are "CLOSED" for business and that we are teetering on the brink of implosion. Our friends and family better run and hide if they don't want to get sucked into our vortex of glandular insanity. Pimples are the last thing we want to contend with when we are not at our best; we don't feel our best and now we don't look our best, either. Kick us when we're down, oh infernal infliction of hormonal Hades. But don't despair our downtrodden Delilah's. Your esthetician is here to explain what you can do to calm down those hormonal breakouts and show your skin who's boss.

Hormonal flare-ups are typically because of a rise in androgen levels. Androgens are a class of steroid hormones. The name "androgen," that means "man," gives us a clue to what these hormones are primarily doing, making men... well, *men*. Androgens give them all their manly characteristics such as a hairy body, deep voice, increased sex drive, less fat, more muscle, aggressive behavior, and oh yeah, testes and a penis. Interesting note: they also help to protect them from depression[10] and negative effects of social isolation[11]. Women's levels of androgens are about one-twelfth that of men. In women, about half of the production of androgen comes from the ovaries in the form of testosterone and androstenedione. The rest come from the adrenal glands mostly as DHEA, which is converted into testosterone and androstenedione primarily in your skin and fat cells, bettcha didn't know your skin and the fat on your ass could do something so wondrous! The biochemical pathways influenced by our androgens are vast and complex and their effect on muscles, skin, gastrointestinal tract, genitourinary tract, bone, brain, cardiovascular system, placenta, and fat tissues are not completely understood.[12][13]

For women, hormone fluctuations involving androgens can cause acne throughout life in association with the following situations:

- Puberty

- Menstruation

- Polycystic ovary syndrome (PCOS)

- Menopause

- Increased androgen levels (for whatever reason, including the use of prescribed testosterone and DHEA)

During puberty, our hormones soar including our androgens, such as testosterone. The rise in androgens triggers higher oil production, especially in the T-zone: the forehead, nose and chin. It also creates changes in cell activity and creates an environment conducive to inflammation, hair follicles clogged with skin cells, and colonization of the clogged follicles by *P. acnes* bacteria, the microbe that prompts pimple parties.

Menstrual acne, the flare-up that coincides with our hormone cycle, is quite common. A study published in the Archives of Dermatology revealed that 63% of women have a premenstrual 25% increase in acne. [14] A menstrual cycle is typically 28 days and every single one of those days is a unique hormone experience. And men call us moody. Well hell yes, we are. We have 28 different moods and we switch them up on a daily basis. No apologies necessary.

Menstruation creates peaks and valleys of hormone levels, with the hormone dominance being estrogen for the first half and progesterone for the second half. Testosterone levels stay about the same. So, when estrogen declines, you become androgen dominant, increasing oil production.

Then when progesterone peaks,
another interesting thing happens,
the pores contract!

Right?! If you ever thought that your pores look smaller on some days while on others, you'd swear that they were trying out for the title of "Crater National Monument", you are not hallucinating. This combination of more oil and tight pores gives some lucky gals a gorgeous glow. But for most of us this leads to congestion and acne. The breakouts typically happen around days 7-10 of the cycle and disappear with the arrival of Aunt Flow.

Polycystic ovary syndrome (PCOS) or Stein-Leventhal syndrome, is a disorder in women that is characterized by an elevated level of male hormones (androgens) and infrequent or absent ovulation (anovulation). A primary trigger for PCOS is obesity, but even if you do not have PCOS, extra weight can still cause flare-ups. To find out how being overweight and eating sugar triggers hormonal breakouts, go read the chapter "Your Weight is Over."

Menopause is like the reverse
of puberty but often delivers
similar outcomes.

According to the American Academy of Dermatology Association, more women in their 30s, 40s, 50s and beyond are experiencing acne. When estrogen levels dip, our androgens start to become more dominant, possibly leading to acne flares. But instead of appearing in the typical T-zone, these pesky pimples appear on the jawline, chin and neck.

As estheticians, we agree with the Dermatology Association as we are seeing more adult acne, especially menopausal acne, and have got to wonder if it is our crazy American lifestyle. Most women we encounter with adult acne also have extremely stressful lives. With overextension comes exhaustion, poor eating habits, lack of exercise and a rise in the numbers on the scale. Carbohydrate heavy diets and inflammatory foods can cause insulin to surge, messing with the delicate balance between estrogen and testosterone. Insulin triggers cells in the ovaries to produce testosterone, which aggravates acne and may produce ruddy skin and unwanted facial hair.

When women enter perimenopause and menopause, the ovaries slow their production of hormones, and the adrenal glands normally pick up the slack and carry us gracefully through the change. Unfortunately, because of our lifestyle, many of us have fatigued adrenals. This will affect how well our glands are going to carry us through menopause. When our adrenals are overworked, they are just too pooped to rise to this challenge. Pronounced morning fatigue may be a tip-off that your adrenals are not working at full capacity and are contributing to menopausal discomfort.

In addition to fatigue, many experience mania (oh, the irony) and spiked anxiety. Xanax, Valium, Ativan and Klonopin have become our crutches to stay calm and get some much-needed sleep... with horrifying outcomes. The use of these highly addictive benzodiazepines is reaching epidemic proportions in the United States with 13.5 million prescriptions written in 2013[15]. Adult acne, obesity, stress, early onset menopause (often with debilitating symptoms including insomnia) and benzo addiction... could there possibly be a connection? We're not rocket scientists, but come on people, think. Think.

If all of this sounds familiar, we are giving you permission to have that "mid-life crisis" in a healthy and constructive way. Maybe it's time to stop and examine your life and ask yourself some interesting questions. Could a move to a different (less expensive) part of the country reduce stress and improve your quality of life? Could you reduce your commute? Meditate instead of medicate? Would you put down your phone and pick up some weights, or a guitar, or a friend to go hiking? Yes, this goes back to hormonal acne because these breakouts are systemic and yes, we are going to give you some tips on how to deal with them, but the real change needs to come from within. Therefore, the first systemic solution suggestion is to reduce stress, stay at a healthy weight and exercise! Other systemic solutions involve drugs, so we recommend you start with self-examination, reinvention and some topical acne aids. It's not easy, but you've only got one life, cherish it.

We offer topical solutions throughout this book. Start with washing your face with a quality cleanser, and when treating acne, avoid harsh scrubs. **Pharmaskincare® Botanica Vit Complex Exfoliant** is a cleanser/exfoliant that does an excellent job of removing excess oil and debris, while gently exfoliating and treating with salicylic acid. Ease into the use of this miracle worker using it 3-4 times per week to begin. This product comes highly recommended, as half of LA is using it to ward off breakouts. Remember your go-to pimple pulverizers as a teenager, Oxy10® and Clearasil®? Good ol' benzoyl peroxide is still the #1 topical to blast acne. 5% works just as well as the 10% and is less drying and irritating. Try to spot treat directly on the problem child for the aforementioned reasons.

For a topical and systemic hormonal-specific acne buster, keep your eyes peeled for phytoestrogens. "Phyto" in Greek means "plant" and the root of "estrogen" which is "estrus" means "sexual desire". Side note: looky here men, when menopause hits, estrogen or "estrus" plummets and guess what, so can a woman's sexual desire. We used to get a break towards the end of our life after we endured endless cramping periods, mood swings, giving birth and raising children (many of us single-handedly, even if a "partner" was hanging around). Then, we finally get to go through menopause, a natural time in our storyline to pause, reflect on life and focus on turning inward, creating from our soul instead of our sexual organs, and possibly, deeply exploring our spirituality in preparation for the "final transition" into the Universal Holiness. And then one day, BAM!, some bastard invents Viagra® and there is no more retiring from the naturally subsiding sexual phase of our life. But that topic warrants another book.

So meanwhile, we are on an eternal quest for the Holy Grail of youth, sexual prowess, and beauty. Circle back to phytoestrogen. They were first observed in 1926, but at that time, it was unknown if they could have an effect on humans and other animals. Until in the 1940s and 1950s, when a herd of sheep in Western Australia were having a hard time getting knocked up[16]. And if that wasn't weird enough, the young maiden sheep had big udders and were sometimes secreting milk! There were some other herds around experiencing the same breeding barriers. The thing they had in common? They were all grazing on the locally developed Dwalganup strain of early subterranean clover and red clover. It was discovered these clovers contained molecules that were acting like "keys" on estrogen receptors[17] and may also modulate the availability of self-produced estrogen[18]. So essentially, these clovers were acting like "the pill" for these female sheep! It's been theorized that plants produce phytoestrogen to control the population size of herbivores[19]! Less baby sheep around, fewer animals devouring all the clover. Clearly, it would be in the best interest of the clover to limit the sheep population. There's Mother Nature again, keeping everything in balance.

Phytoestrogens are a type of xenoestrogen, a synthetic or natural chemical that mimics estrogen. Naturally occurring phytoestrogens are found in flax, nuts and nut butters, soybeans, sunflower seeds, yams, apples, beer, garbanzo beans (mmmmm... hummus), red clover and many, many more plants. But don't worry, consuming these foods will not throw us into a state of infertility like the sheep. Our digestive system is completely different from theirs, rendering a milder outcome.

But for women going through menopause, these plants sound like miracle workers with the promise of acting like a food-based estrogen replacement, increasing metabolism, reducing insulin surges, and possibly decreasing perimenopause and menopause symptoms. And even though a wide range of beneficial effects of phytoestrogens have been claimed, such as a reduction in risk of cancer and postmenopausal symptoms and an increase in cardiovascular, central nervous system and metabolic health, there is also concern that they may act as endocrine disrupters and adversely affect our wellness. Right now, based on available evidence, it's just not clear[20]. Most clinical trials detected no significant effects on classic menopausal symptoms. Soy seems to be the best bet and can help with certain aspects, such as sleep disturbances and mood swings, but the level of relief is low to none. The <u>topical</u> use of phytoestrogens may present a "happy medium" for balancing benefits without excessive systemic exposure.

Our collagen production does not happen to *randomly* correlate perfectly with our estrogen production. No, no, they are indeed linked with estrogen stimulating collagen; both peaking at our tender age of 27. Ahhh... the "firm years". A study on the decrease of skin collagen in postmenopausal women found a decrease of 2.1 percent per year in the first fifteen years post-menopause. On average, from age fifty to sixty-five, more than 30 percent of collagen will be lost due to the cessation of estrogen. Loss of collagen, skin's source of strength and elasticity, aggravates sagging, wrinkling, and thinning of skin[21].

Lucky for us there are estrogen receptors in our skin, particularly our facial skin, and phytoestrogens can pass through the skin and act as "keys" to unlock the receptors stimulating not only higher collagen production but increased hyaluronic acid production, improved photo-protection, wound healing and protection against oxidative stress, breakouts and unwanted hair.

There's a product line out that we love to love called **VENeffect**® created by chicks (an OB/GYN and her sister, a beauty expert) *for* chicks. They packed their products full of phytoestrogens, such as resveratrol, and extracts from pomegranate, willow bark, and red clover, of course! The aim of the creators of these products was to "balance out hormones right in the epidermis and dermis for gorgeous, glowing, and clear skin."

Tanis' & Neddy's Sidebar: Synthetic Xenoestrogens

In our modern world, plants are not the only sources of xenoestrogens, and they are not all created equal. Synthetic xenoestrogens are ubiquitous in our environment and pose substantial health risks. They have similar effects as phytoestrogens, making it difficult to separate out the actions of these agents during population studies[22]. But this we do know; excessive synthetic xenoestrogens in our environment are having deleterious effects. They are endocrine system disruptors leading to several developmental abnormalities in humans and wildlife.

Some of the greatest effects of xenoestrogens happen on humans during puberty; a critical time for sexual differentiation. The effects of these agents can lead to precocious puberty (PP). Precocious puberty is when a child's body changes into an adult too soon. Puberty, that begins before the age of eight in girls and nine in boys, is PP, and it's on the rise. The normal age used to be 15 for the onset of puberty and now it's occurring at seven, eight and nine years old! Scientists agree PP is dramatically increasing, but the jury is still out on the exact cause. They have definitively linked to xenoestrogens in the environment[23] but the other culprit may be obesity. The extra calories and the protein leptin, produced in fatty tissue, tell the brain that clearly, there's plenty of food around and it's safe to reproduce and a biochemical cascade triggers puberty. This is not a healthy "new normal" for our children.

Here are a few common synthetic xenoestrogens and where they are found:

- **Atrazine** this is the most heavily used herbicide in the US used to kill weeds. It's used on sugarcane, corn, hay and winter wheat crops and is applied to Christmas trees, golf courses, lawns and recreational areas where our children play.

- **BPA** Bisphenol A is used to manufacture plastics and resins and is one of the highest volume produced chemicals worldwide[24]. It lines most food and beverage containers and might cause disease in humans[25]. Step away from the can opener...

- **Dioxin** these highly toxic chemicals are released in smoke when things like wood, trash, coal, oil and that cigarette hanging out the side of your mouth are burned and when papers and wood pulps are bleached white using chlorine. Dioxin gets into the environment when the smoke settles on agricultural fields or where livestock graze and when fish ingest it through contaminated water supplies. It loves to hang out in fat and more than 90% of human exposure is through eating fatty food such as meat (including fish and shellfish) and dairy. Then it hangs out in our fat for up to 11 years and is slow to release[26]. Dioxin affects breast tissue and is linked to the inability to breastfeed offspring[27] and cancer[28].

- **Endosulfan** is an insecticide used on fruits, vegetables, grains and trees. We are exposed when we eat foods treated with this insecticide or when we are exposed to groundwater contaminated with it.

- **Phthalates** give plastics such as polyvinyl chloride flexibility and can be found in floorings, medical devices and wall coverings. Phthalates are also found in lotions, perfumes, cosmetics, varnishes and in the coating of time-released medications.

- **Zeranol** this is an anabolic growth promoter used to fatten up livestock in the US and Canada.

There are many more and Wikipedia will give you a decent list so you can search them out in everything from your food, to its containers, to your toiletries, and your everyday plastics. For advice on how to clean up xenoestrogens from your child's and your environment, check out Dr. Mercola's website at www.drmercola.com.

There are systemic solutions for hormonal breakouts that are different than eating foods with xenoestrogens. An interesting plant-based solution involves the ingestion of peppermint. Botanists believe it is a hybrid of spearmint and watermint with menthol and methone being its two primary active agents. This oil was being used by all the hip ancients including the Egyptians, Japanese, Chinese, and Greeks, and is one of the oldest European herbs used for medicinal purposes.

Peppermint persists in our population because it helps alleviate so many ailments! We took a little count and found at least 50 different uses and benefits ranging from diminishing nausea to reducing breastfeeding discomfort to protecting against Alzheimer's and cancer.

In a study published in Phytomedicine, peppermint oil had the same headache soothing effects as 1000mg of acetaminophen. When combined with eucalyptus oil, use increases cognitive abilities while relaxing muscles and mind[29]. Trust us, we diffused a lot of these two oils while writing this book. Peppermint oil, particularly in combination with other essential oils (e.o.) Such as fennel, sage, clary sage and lavender can help balance hormones in women. This blend helps increase estrogen levels and decrease testosterone levels in women, and it can naturally enhance fertility and relieve PMS symptoms.

Peppermint can also relieve the symptoms of polycystic ovarian syndrome (PCOS) in two ways. First, drinking peppermint tea helps alleviate depression, acne (more on this in a minute), masculine patterns of hair growth, along with other masculinizing symptoms, and infertility. Second, peppermint supports weight loss, and weight loss is key to not only reducing the symptoms of PCOS but also curing it. A study published in the International Journal of Obesity reported that inhaling peppermint oil affected the satiety center of the hypothalamus. Over 3,000 people took part in this study and the average weight loss was 30 pounds just from sniffin' mint![30]

And if all that wasn't enough. Peppermint tea can give a slight estrogen boost to some drinkers, which will help curb hormonal hiccups and also clear hormonal acne! We've had clients consistently use 1-2 drops of e.o. in a glass of water during the day and then drink peppermint tea at night with positive outcomes; fewer breakouts and less inflammation! And with that cup of tea before bed, you may enjoy the added benefit of more restful sleep. This is like Mother Nature throwing women a bone. She has supplied us with this amazing herb that aids with so many chick-related challenges, so be a Peppermint Pattie and get the kettle on!

Tanis' & Neddy's Sidebar: Using Essential Oils

The receptors in the human nose can discern over a trillion distinct smells! When Tanis was working at Kraft and Anhueser-Busch, they taught her how to sniff out yeast cells in liquids and how to pick up on the different odor characteristics in water, distinguishing well water from spring from city from reverse osmosis water. Yes, our noses are that sensitive! When airborne molecules connect with the cilia in our nose, the olfactory cells produce a nerve impulse which reaches the Limbic System, one of the most primitive parts of our brain concerned with emotions and survival. The activity of the nerve signals passing through Limbic Land causes mood changes by altering the brain's chemistry. Our body is responding to the aroma even before our brain recognizes and names it!

Essential oils also communicate with the hippocampus and amygdala in the brain, the key areas that store emotions and memories. Makes sense that smells are the #1 trigger for our feelings and reminiscing! Think of a time a smell has reminded you of something like a favorite place or person. Does Polo cologne conjure up any feelings? How about the smell of pine trees or a cedar closet? Ever go into a house for sale and they've got the cinnamon and vanilla wafting through the air? Makes you *feel* pretty cozy, right? Tanis' real estate agent sold her house in eight days... could the freshly baking cookies in the oven have had something to do with it? When e.o.s is inhaled, our mood, blood pressure, sleep, motivation, heart rate and stress levels is altered.

Essential oils also support the control center of the brain, the hypothalamus, that regulates body temperature, hunger, thirst, sleep, mood, and sex drive. It sends messages to your adrenals, pituitary, thyroid and endocrine system (including your sex organs) and regulates hunger and thirst impulses and your ability to handle stress. Therefore, during menopause, when estrogen levels are fluctuating, the hypothalamus becomes confused and, like a cell phone with a poor connection, it cannot get the proper signals out to the rest of your body. The estrogen flux causes the hypothalamus to send out faulty messages and one of those is telling your system that there are temperature changes in your body, when actually, there are not. Hot flashes and cold flashes in addition to other challenges due to wacked-out hypothalamus communications, such as insomnia, mood swings, and hunger, thirst and sex impulses gone wild, can be addressed by talking to your hypothalamus. And what better way to have a chat with the brain center than through the use of essential oils?! We rely on Young Living® e.o.s because we know they are high quality, pure, organic, and food-grade. They have single note oils and blends made for specific outcomes such as Clarity™, EN-R-GEE™, Stress Away™, and Dragon Time™ (yeah, for that "special" time of the month or whenever you feel like breathing fire).

Another systemic remedy for hormonal breakouts is... how shall we put this... hormones! We know that dabbling in hormone-therapy whether it be birth control pills, spironolactone, or the ever more popular bio-identical hormone replacement therapy (HRT) is a big decision that you and your doctor need to make as a team. We can briefly explain some options and how they work in combating breakouts.

- **Birth control pills** The pill, increases a protein called sex-hormone binding globulin which acts like a testosterone sponge. When the ratio of estrogen to testosterone increases, the effects of testosterone, including breakouts, decrease. The pill can also slow down oil production. Some pills specifically approved to manage acne are Ortho Tri-Cyclen®, Estrosten®, and Yaz®. Be patient. It takes your body a few months to adjust to the new hormones and sometimes acne will stay the same or worsen before it subsides.

- **Spironolactone** This is a cardiovascular drug that also acts as an "androgen-blocker". If acne is unresponsive to other treatments, a doctor may consider this treatment for you.

- **Bio-identical HRT** This is for women who have started to go through the change either very early in life (say 40) and/or they are having a hell of a time with it. First, you need to pick up a copy of the book The Hormone Decision by Tara Parker-Pope[31]. She gives you the pros and cons and breaks down the data so you can start your own contemplation process. Second, you need to find a doctor that has A LOT of experience with HRT. There is a science and an art to this therapy. They will discuss all the benefits and all the risks with you. Then, you really need to do your homework, some deep soul searching, and heed the advice of your physician before deciding. The treatment begins with an in-depth profile of your current hormone levels. It should include blood, urine and saliva testing; most or all of which will *not* be covered by your insurance. Then customized creams and pills are made just for you at a compounding pharmacy, which are also *not* paid for by your insurance. Viagra® *is* covered, on the other hand, because clearly, not getting a boner is a life-threatening situation. HRT is *not* covered, because after all, menopause symptoms are all in our heads, right? We digress. Then, after you begin, you will need to continue to monitor your hormones and your doctor will make adjustments as needed. Sounds like a lot of time, money and trouble? Yes, it is. It's a huge expense, pain in the ass and can include risks. And women are still doing it. That's how hellacious menopause can be. Tanis thinks it's worth every penny.

WHAT YOUR ESTHETICIAN REALLY WANTED TO TELL YOU

- Androgen dominance can mean hormonal breakouts. Androgen dominance can occur during puberty, at certain times in the menstrual cycle and during menopause.

- Reducing stress, increasing exercise, eating a healthy plant-based diet and reducing your household load of synthetic xenoestrogens can help support balanced hormones, leading to vitality and clear, gorgeous skin!

- Phytoestrogens can work both systemically and topically to mimic estrogen and possibly relieve some menopausal symptoms.

- There are myriad of both topical and systemic remedies that can help ward off hormonal breakouts. Talk to your esthetician and doctor and ask for guidance.

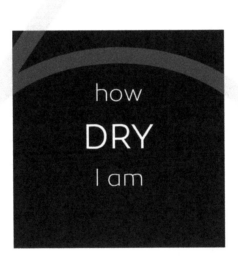

how
DRY
I am

6

HOW DRY I AM

SWEAT OR SUFFER

Sweat it out. When in doubt, go to the Korean Day Spa. Buy at least 10 entry passes and then make up every excuse on the planet to get your naked butt in there at least a few times per month. If you are one of our facial clients, and you are breaking out, there is *no doubt* we have asked you if you exercise, take hot baths, sauna, speak in front of large groups of people, or are in menopause; basically, if you profusely perspire. Sweating helps to boost the immune system, flush out excess salt, reduce the chance of kidney stones, and keeps you from overheating. Sweat helps you get rid of crap in your body. Like Tanis' bro', Tom often says, "Dilution is the Solution for the Pollution".

And with that being said, sweating, especially heavy, will cause you to lose water and electrolytes, so for all of this to be beneficial, please drink, drink, drink. Two to three liters to be precise. Freshly tapped coconut water (www.cocotaps.com), alkaline water or just plain filtered spring water are our beverages of choice. And remember, some of the heating (and cooling) practices described in this chapter are cultural conventions that begin at an early age and are guided by experienced elders, so *always* consult with your physician before trying out new wellness regimes.

Sweat Prep-Work: We always recommend that if you have not broken a heavy sweat in a few months, and you have not been extracted by a licensed esthetician in a while, start with extractions. Those big old plugs of oxidized, solidified oil, salt and dirt are like giant boulders that need to be removed from the stream before the river runs through it. You think they are going to gently lift out with a Biore® strip? Think again, my little friend. They are going to have to be evicted with substantial force and conviction and skill, possibly a jack hammer, electric drill and blasted out with a small amount of TNT. Ok, we're just kidding (sort of) but if they have been lodged in there for months, years, decades, you know it is going to take a tenacious, highly experienced professional, working under a magnifying lamp to get them out.

Next, hit the gym, jump some rope, steam in the sauna or soak in a hot tub (preferably with a few naked models) but do something. Do ANYTHING to dump a deluge. And if you haven't done so already, please go read the chapter entitled "It's a Workout – not Tinder". 'Nuf said. So now you have received a professional facial, washed your face, opened the floodgates and pushed all that dirt, excess oil, salt and bacteria onto the surface of your skin. Now what? Better go read the chapter "Wash Your F*cking Face". Oh, I'm sorry, does this sound like a lot of work? Then keep your pimpled up, drab, dull, and lifeless complexion and stop bitching about your less-than-looks. Just sayin'. You want your cheeks to be clear and glowing like a newborn's butt? Then work for it, baby.

Perspiration Perks: There are so many benefits to perspiration that we are going to lay them out for you in case we haven't convinced you to strip naked and sweat:

- **Blast Bacteria**: Dermcidin, an antimicrobial protein that prevents the proliferation of *P. acnes*, is commonly found, guess where? Yup, in human sweat! Dermcidin reduces this bad bacteria's ability to create RNA and proteins necessary for survival [32][33]. Research has also revealed that patients with acne had a significantly lower amount of this *P. acnes* pulverizing protein in their sweat[34]. But even if you run low on dermcidin, there is still another solution.

- **A Salty Solution**: The salt in your sweat is also toxic to these naughty bacteria. And with increased circulation and hydration [35] from your self-induced saunic heat wave, the healing times of any pimple party boo-boos will most likely decrease while the moisture content of your stratum corneum, the most top layer of your skin, should increase. Plump, clear, glowing, balanced skin. Win, win, win, and win.

- **Purge Pores**: Sweat also washes out all that clogged up debris hanging out in your pores. While simultaneously warming the skin, it allows excess oil to be flushed out when it is still in the liquid state.

- **Toxic Clean Up**: Sweating helps you eliminate phthalates, sometimes more than twice as much as is pissed out through your urine[36]. Phthalates are a common and risky ingredient in personal care products and are so ubiquitous that they are darn near impossible to avoid. Eyelash glue, phthalates. Fragrance, phthalates. New car smell? Yup, phthalates. But these are a few of our favorite things! Sigh, better go sweat.

- **Heavy Metal Removal**: Perspiration helps purge the heavy stuff, as in metals, such as mercury and arsenic and lead oh my[37]!

Although there are myriad ways to sweat, the traditional sauna can be traced back to Finland and may have originated as early as 7,000 BC! It's like an oven that heats you from the outside in. Our clients also ask us about infrared saunas which heat from the inside out, but yield similar results, so either sauna will do a body good.

Benefits of Sauna: No surprise that the first sauna-skin study analyzed the regular use of a traditional Finnish sauna's effect on skin versus not partaking at all. Here's some convincing data to shack up and sweat:

1) Sauna contributes to changes in skin pH regulation[33]. A drop in the skin's pH observed with sauna could strengthen the skin's acid mantle, creating a more acidic environment, making it more difficult for *P. acnes* to grow (compared to the other bacteria on the skin)[33][34]. *P. acnes* being the main bacterial beastie for creating zits.

2) Measurements taken of participants' skin demonstrated that regular sauna reduces skin sebum production as measured from the forehead [32].

3) Saunas increase your energy expenditure and calories burned. A dry sauna burns more calories than a hot bath; you're looking at about 300-500 calories per 30-minute session [38].

4) Saunas increase secretion of the human growth hormone [39] (the *real* fountain of youth).

5) Saunas help to lower total cholesterol and LDL (the "bad" component of cholesterol) similar to moderate-intensity physical exercise [40]! If you made it to the gym, but you're too lazy to exercise, go sit in the sauna.

6) As your core temperature rises, so does your immune system [41]. Get hot and watch your number of colds be reduced to almost half [42]. Just don't share a steam room with a sick buddy (viruses are carried on water droplets).

7) Sauna before counting sheep to get better sleep [43]! The people of Finland reported that sauna was right up there not far behind regular exercise and reading/listening to music to lull them off to slumberland. Baaa.

Sauna Bonus-Up: Now for the pièce de résistance, saunas increase your metabolism! Research confirms that getting hot (sauna, steam room, hot tub), not looking hot, after a workout not only ramps up calorie burn but has a beneficial effect on blood sugar levels. A study conducted by exercise physiologist Steve Faulkner, PhD showed that soaking in a tub of water at 104 degrees Fahrenheit for one hour increased energy output by 80% and burned 140 calories per hour; comparable to a brisk 30-minute walk. Who wouldn't rather soak than walk! They also tested the participants' blood glucose level after eating a meal and then soaking or exercising for one hour. The bathers had a 10% lower post-meal glucose level than the exercisers, probably due to heat shock proteins released when, well, you get really freakin' hot! Shocking, we know. They probably move the glucose out of the blood and into your skeletal muscle, reducing blood sugar levels and improving insulin sensitivity [44]. We love to exercise, eat, soak, then sleep. Yes, in that exact order. An amazing way to end the day and so much more beneficial and rewarding than the telly, we think.

Cryotherapy Considerations: So as not to be biased towards just thermic spa activities, we must give our frosty frolics some page space, too. Bread and butter, Kim and Kanye, pickles and peanut butter; some things are inseparable, including sauna and cold plunge. Full circle back to the Korean jimjilbang. Look around. See all that tight, youthful looking Korean skin? See the toddlers that are there learning the ancient techniques of exfoliation, vasodilation, and masking with snail trail? Yup, most Koreans have early memories of partaking of the sauna followed by the cold plunge followed by the sauna followed by the cold plunge; the yin and yang of the bathhouse experience. Taking the gelid dunk has its own set of health and beauty benefits, including reducing fatigue from chronic-fatigue syndrome [45] (if dunking into ice water doesn't jolt you into motion, what the hell will?). It also increases calorie burning [46], boosts immunity [47], improves glucose tolerance and enhances the insulin response [48].

It also activates your brown adipose tissue (BAT) that melts away the evil white fat [49]. The higher your BAT, the lower your fat! Getting chilly also helps reduce your food cravings. We agree as we find it damn near impossible to stuff our face with frigid fingers.

Full water submersion in icy temps is a learned art, as Tanis will tell you. She has been practicing for over a decade and on a good day, may even impress her fellow K spa attendees with extended periods in the snow zone. And why not when the benefits to skin are instantaneous.

Cold plunging instantly tightens
pores slowing oil production and
helps to de-puff tissue.

The experience goes something like this and can vary from person to person:

1) Your body realizes it just got colder than a witch's titty and the blood vessels on your extremities constrict. This slows heat loss and also allows the blood to hang out more near the vital organs like your heart and your brain (vital to most, but the more we read beauty blogs we realize not vital to all). This protects the two main powerhouses of the body.

2) After about five to ten minutes of cold exposure, the blood vessels in the extremities and skin suddenly vasodilate, flushing the tissue with blood and warmth. This can feel interesting to say the least and is sometimes called the "hot aches" (also brought on by looking at photos of David Kimmerle). You end up looking like a lobster at a Maine beach picnic, but it is only a temporary effect, the benefits however, are worth it!

Tanis swears polar plunging helped save her very broken leg with astonishing healing rates and results. We are swearing by the jimjilbang at $15 for the day; seaweed soup and snail trail mask not included.

Not into icy hydro-adventures? Then you can jump onto the cryotherapy bandwagon like Kobe Bryant. In body cryotherapy, you stand in a chamber cooled with liquid nitrogen (with your head outside of the chamber) or a room cooled by electricity (this is the preferred method – head included) with temperatures as low as minus 200°F. You didn't think you could get in a room that crazy cold – did you? Neither did we… until one day we leaped into icicle land and we never wanted to leave. Well actually, about 2.5 minutes later we were pushing each other over trying to get out of the f*cking door, but you get the idea.

The cost is anywhere from $20 to $90 a hit. We recently discovered USCryotherapy® and purchased a very affordable monthly unlimited pass. Can we just say that we are addicted and think that our joints have never felt better and our skin has never looked quite so good if we do say so ourselves! We love posting selfies looking like "Girls Gone Wild – the Iceland Edition" on our IG page (taken by friends holding cameras *outside* of the glacier chamber, BTW don't be a *pendeja* and bring your phone into the steam room or sauna either). It's great for reducing inflammation after an intense workout, to jumpstart your day, or if you are in desperate need, like us, for social media material. Happy Snappy!

WHAT YOUR ESTHETICIAN **REALLY** WANTED TO TELL YOU

- Sweat profusely at least three times per week, we suggest six or seven.

- Drink liters of water each day, two to three, to be precise.

- Get extractions and wash your face *before* sweating.

- Buy passes to your favorite Korean Day Spa. Entry should be between $10 - $20. If you do not live near a Korean Day Spa, move.

what's my

ADRENALS

gotta do with it

?

7

WHAT'S MY ADRENALS GOTTA DO WITH IT?

EVERYTHING

When we hear the word addiction, things like alcohol, drugs, sex, cigarettes, gambling and, yes, even shopping may come to mind. But it seems living in the age of lightning-fast communications, information, distractions and pleasures, primarily based on the use of smartphones, have created another deceptive addiction that hurts people's families, work performance and satisfaction, their health and their skin. It is the addiction to adrenaline. And these days, it's not just executives that are vulnerable to life at full throttle; many are convinced that anything slower represents lost opportunities, lost experiences and lost income.

Neddy recently worked on a 13-year-old boy's skin, let's call him Angel, who was breaking out. Yes, he's facing a full-blown eruption of puberty at any second and his skin is teetering on the edge of childhood hormone levels to those of King Kong on testosterone crack, but the surprise was when he said his number one concern was stress. Pressure to perform well in school with workloads sometimes mimicking that found on college campuses, in addition to, being involved in sports and as a community leader so he will be able to get into a school that will get him into the next school that will get him into that internship that will get him into that job that will get him into that divorce court that will get him into that rehab center.

Unlike other addictions, adrenaline junkies are often praised for their coffee swilling lifestyles frantically working, exercising, and parenting their way to the top of their careers, Zumba class and PTA Board. The dopamine and adrenaline rush that accompanies stressful lifestyles can become addictive and the addict can unconsciously encourage this elevated state of hormones by overpacking schedules, engaging in unnecessary arguments and risky behaviors all while packing in five or more days of strenuous exercise in the name of good health.

And what happens when your cell phone stops pinging for two whole minutes or you go on vacation and God forbid it's in a location without reception (do they even exist)? Your brain tells you it's bored and tries to create a situation to get its next adrenaline hit. Huzzah for that Starbucks® where you just guzzled a Plus 2X Caffeine coffee and where the dude in the parking lot just stole your space, they are both helping you to get your adrenaline fix. Excuse me, your addiction is beginning to show on your skin.

When stressed or consuming caffeine or our Western World fave doing both simultaneously because more is always better, your adrenal glands, that sit atop your kidneys release a surge of hormones including adrenaline and cortisol. These hormones increase your heart rate, elevate your blood pressure, and increase energy. Wow! kind of like a first kiss. Now doesn't that feel good?! Uh Huh! But wait, there's more. This hormone burst also sets off an inflammatory cascade in the body with amazing and life altering side effects such as weight gain, gastrointestinal distress, a slew of diseases including the big C, adrenal fatigue (Google it) and for the icing; adult acne, eczema, wrinkles and, well, premature aging. So that is why we are constantly asked as estheticians: "why do I have pimples and wrinkles at the same time?" Put down the phone and the latte and let's talk.

First, seek support. Adrenaline addiction is being treated as a serious disorder and you can get help through individual counseling or even at addiction treatment centers. Step one is to recognize the problem and proudly declare you are about to kick it in the ass. Then seek professional help and turn your life into the Zen Zone that you can daringly create.

Second, go read "Confessions of an Adrenaline Addict" by Adoley Odunton and Deborah Deras [50]. In it, Odunton and Deras confess to the destructive nature of their own adrenaline addictions and give step-by-step advice on how to recover and create a life of ease and grace. Third, think positive. This helps to calm your crazy adrenals and, according to an Olay® study, also seems to be the secret weapon of "Super Agers" women who look 10 or more years younger than their actual age. Positively Fabulous!

Seven more things to reduce stress and age less:

1) Work out! 'nuf said.

2) Hug a tree, get outside and be in nature.

3) Get real, realistic people are often happy people.

4) Meditate.

5) Use music to reduce stress. In a study conducted in Switzerland, listening to classical music before being exposed to a stressful stimulus significantly reduced the stress response, including cortisol secretion, in 60 healthy females [51].

6) Try Neurofeedback. Caring individuals at The Sleep Recovery Center will set you up to conduct 50-minute treatments in the comfort of *your own home* that tell your brain to calm the f*ck down. Individuals have found it to radically reduce anxiety, stress eating, combative behavior, and freaking out while increasing focus, sleep, and feelings of peace. www.sleeprecoverycenters.com

7) Get off of social media. It was made to connect us, but common outcomes are feelings of anxiety and competition. Even better, get off of your phone completely. Many of us grab our phones

an *extra* 100 times per day more than we should. Try using your phone to keep off of your phone! Check out the "Forest" app. Open it up when you are focusing on an offline task. If you don't touch your phone, your virtual tree grows and grows! If you leave the app to burn time on FB or post your latest selfie on IG, your tree kicks the bucket. Be a good forest ranger and you earn "coins" which are used to plant plants through the Trees for the Future nonprofit org. Or try this… a 24-hour monthly retreat with no electronics, no talking, no reading (not even this stupendous book), yeah, no shit. You will feel better and look awesome doing it!

Back to Angel. His very conscious parents decided _not_ to give Angel a smartphone, tablet, X-box, etc. and Angel understands that it's in his best interest to reduce distractions in order to reduce stress. He is currently thriving in school, both intellectually and socially, even though he is an electronic-free individual. Perhaps one day Angel will also be a "Super Ager"… but for now he's satisfied with being "Super Angel". Om yes!

WHAT YOUR ESTHETICIAN **REALLY** WANTED TO TELL YOU

- This is bigger than esthetics and as weighty as the "Your Weight is Over" chapter. We see it in your skin and we are so concerned that stress can ruin your skin, your life, and can even kill. Please don't ask us for lotions and potions. We want to give you real help. Examine your life and your children's lives and ask those hard questions. Maybe those questions are going to require tough answers, but we have faith in you. Seek relief.

- Remember, your skin is like a monitor, you need to watch it as much as you watch your smartphone, telly, tablet, computer…

whatever, whatever. Unlike those distracters showing you what you want to see... your skin is showing you what you NEED to see. Take off your blindfold. Stay woke.

- Cut caffeine. Go herbal.

- Don't worry, be happy.

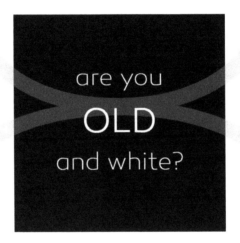

8

ARE YOU OLD AND WHITE?

STOP OVER-MOISTURIZING

We remember reading somewhere in esthetician school that perfectly healthy and balanced skin needs no moisturizer. Perhaps there is some truth in that, but until we reach the epitome, the nonpareil, the ne plus ultra, the ultimate and most high state of skin perfection, bring it. Especially for old white women. But if "black don't crack" seems like it best describes you or you are under the age of 50 and you are piling on the cream, put yourself on pause. Let's examine ethnic stereotypes, oil versus water dryness, and other factors that affect the succulence of your stratum corneum. Then you can decide if you need to put down and walk away from the moisturizer.

Is darker skin really more oily, and hydrated? Black skin has more casual lipids and more moisture in the stratum corneum than white skin exhibiting as hydrated, smoother, plumper skin. So yes, it is. BTW the amount of sweat glands in black and white skin is identical and varies with climatic changes, but not with racial factors [52]. Also, in darkly pigmented persons, a thicker and more compact dermis makes facial lines less noticeable [53]. Blacks have about twenty cell layers compared to sixteen in whites [52].

Highly pigmented or not; Asian, Native, South American, or Icelandic; are you a person who feels you have a fair share of oil and hydration? Then make sure you are exfoliating to remove excess oil and dead cells to prepare your skin for that lightweight moisturizer you are about to apply. Also recommended are regular (meaning about every 6 weeks) extractions to keep those pores free of solidified oil plugs.

So, there is some truth in that old adage, but what about the thousands of other ethnicities, not to mention the many extrinsic (environmental) and intrinsic (internal) factors affecting the skin? This is when we want you to act like an estie… get up, walk over to the mirror and LOOK at your skin! Do you have congestion, pimples, and blackheads? Do you experience an oily sheen halfway through the day? Does your face get a little itchy after several hours of not cleansing and feel more balanced and calm after a good suds up and scrub down? This means you are probably doing well in the oil production department.

Oily skin does best with a very
light weight moisturizer even if it
is dry from a lack of water.

We recommend drinking a lot of water and sweating (with a clean face, please see the chapter "Wash Your F*cking Face"). The heat generated from exercise and the flow of water through the pores helps to keep the oil in the liquid state and flowing out of the pores and onto the surface of the skin, where it belongs. Just as long as you drink, drink, drink, this will help to simultaneously flush out excess oil *and* hydrate skin. Win–Win.

Again, LOOK at your skin. Are you free of congestion, breakouts, and plugs? Is your skin flaky, itchy, dry or peeling, especially *after* cleansing? Is it crepey under your eyes after you wash? Welcome to the "officially dry" club. Sweating is still a great way to naturally hydrate the skin (remember, this only works if you drink enough water, for us that's 1-3 Liters per day). Then, find a great moisturizer avoiding mineral oil-based creams that are occlusive or ones that have a lot of water and useless filler. Instead, choose one with active ingredients such as peptides, ceramides, hyaluronic acid and botanicals that hydrate and plump. Spot treat if necessary (and it is almost always necessary): a little more around the eyes and mouth, less or none on the T-zone, you get the picture. Remember to apply moisturizer to your neck and décolleté especially the area on the side of the neck that connects to the shoulder. Look in the mirror at these areas. This is where your friend is staring at you during Sunday brunch.

Now, of course, many other intrinsic factors come into play when it comes to hydration, but overall, we see people piling on the potions a little too much. Most skin we work on could use a little extra moisture under the eyes and around the lips where there is the least amount of secretory glands. And of course, we support you if you are using a lotion as a vehicle to apply an active ingredient such as AHA, a retinoid or sunscreen. But if your skin is not visibly dry and flaky, less can be more. We deal with more problems (congestion, milia, breakouts) due to over moisturizing (usually with petrochemical derivative heavy creams) than problems with under moisturizing. And if you are going to moisturize, the best time is after you drink your evening nightcap of water and before drifting off to LaLaLand.

Tanis' & Neddy's Sidebar: The "Oil Cleansing" Trend

O-M-G. We think the person who thought of this trend must have been an estie who needed more business. After the trend broke, we saw a rash (pun intended) of clients who came in because they experienced the most god-awful breakouts, because of product use. Let's be clear, an oil is an oil is an oil and unless you have low oil, dry skin, you need to really think about putting it on your face, especially as a cleanser!

So, who should give oil cleansing a go? Are you dry and old? Going through menopause and your skin is wrinkling up like a prune before your very eyes? Do you have skin on the dry side and are on the run and only want to carry a few products in your travel bag? If you meet any of these criteria for being a good candidate to experiment with oil cleansing, we recommend you stick with a formulation designed to do specifically this (such as **Eminence®** **Stone Crop Cleansing Oil**, which we LOVE). These formulations will most likely have a hydrophobic component (oil loving which clings to the oil and dirt on your skin) and a hydrophilic component (water loving which makes them rinse off more thoroughly with water taking the dirt and oil along for the ride) making them actually function as a cleanser.

Some of the most tragic breakouts we have seen are from attempting to "cleanse" the face with coconut, almond, olive, the ever-so-trendy sea buckthorn oil alone or in conjunction with castor oil. Just because something comes from nature, it doesn't mean you should put it on your skin. And just because some beauty blogger blogged it that doesn't mean it is right for you. And if you have uppity skin and are prone to breakouts and *still* want to try this trend, you can contact us at AskTheEstheticians@gmail.com because you probably are gonna need an estie right quick.

WHAT YOUR ESTHETICIAN
REALLY WANTED TO TELL YOU

- Please buy that high-quality moisturizer from us with all those botanicals and powerful active ingredients, just don't overuse it and make sure the formulation is right for your skin. Your estie needs to ensure this and exchange the product if it is not working for you. If your estie won't do this, they're "Just Not That Into You". Go read the book.

- Look at your skin and spot treat. Think you have combination skin? Skin that changes with the seasons? Of course, you do. Pay attention.

- Be a cream conservationist. Oily, well-hydrated skin? Sure, financially we would love to sell you a boatload of moisturizer but ethically, we know it's a waste of money and very precious resources. Less is more.

- We are not huge fans of moisturizers that are water, mineral oil, or petrochemical derivative based with little to no additional active ingredients for reasons mentioned elsewhere in this book but hey, it's your money.

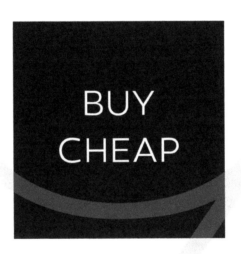

9

BUY CHEAP

BREAK OUT

Ah, ingredients. That long list of components on the back label of everything. Most people skip it, partly because it looks like a foreign language. Or, we simply can't read it because it's so friggin' small (our solution for this is to take a pic with our phone, enlarge the photo, and analyze away). And if looking at ingredients isn't headache inducing enough, imagine doing it on a budget?! Some think they have to bankroll an impeccable clinical grade skin care regimen to have bright and youthful skin. We mean, "Hello, La Mers® of the world!" We've had many thrifty, fiscally savvy clients (bless their hearts) juggle with the anxiety of dropping their hard-earned dinero for these pricey brands. And to this, we command them to "hold your horses!" Is that pricey product stickered with a dollar amount because of its superlative active ingredient list? Or is that cost because they needed to cut a check to Jennifer Aniston or it's toting a label with 2 capital "C"s? And just because you're paying through the nose for a product doesn't mean it comes with a guarantee it will not wreak havoc on your skin. And as for that costly beachy branded product line, this company is known for loading up professional makeup artists (many of which are our friends) with tons of their products, hoping the makeup artist will then introduce them to their movie star client.

More often than not, the products make the celebrity's skin breakout and now the artist has to do overtime covering up a poor decision. It's no surprise (to us) when our clients experience a similar scene because their medicine cabinets and vanities are piled high with pricey, pimple-producing products full of common irritants and comedogenic crap. So, when it comes to price points of products and their performance, is the truth simple? Do we get what we pay for? Should we break the bank in belief that good skin care should be an investment of goliath proportions… or should we just throw in the towel and cruise the aisle of the Dollar King looking for our next anti-aging potion?

In this chapter, we are going to give you some tips and list some ingredients to keep in mind when shopping for products that can work for you on your budget. We are going to hijack your hygiene routine and kick up your knowledge! First things first, so we're on the same page here, let's blow your mind with something that is contrary to common belief, particularly in the beauty blog realm. When it comes to skincare, price and product effectiveness are NOT directly correlated. Gasp! Yes, you heard us! We just typed that out loud. Sure, superior ingredients can be steep. Therefore, one could easily assume that this means the more expensive the product, the better the components, and the more effective it will be. Or vice-versa. But in the beauty industry, this is not always the case. In the words of our cosmetic chemist hero, Perry Romanowski, co-founder of The Beauty Brains, "Price and effectiveness are not equal in the cosmetic industry." Why not? Marketing costs, packaging, and brand affiliation can inflate prices while use of cheap ingredients that increase volume of the product without adding any substantial benefit (known as "fillers") cheapen it.

Think of it this way. Like that affordable bouquet. Yeah, sure there are roses in it, like two. The majority of flowers are "*fillers.*" Cheap yet bulky foliage like baby's breath or leaves off of some random-ass plant that look like they were taken from our yard, fern and the like. The more "filler" the less the aroma and visual impact from the headliners, the roses. Don't get us wrong; it can look nice and pretty all tightly bundled in its wrapper, but stick it in a vase and give it a whiff, and it's a sad situation. What a rip off! This is why a pricey dozen roses is always touted as a big romantic gesture. Now imagine taking that measly bouquet and dangling a Christian Dior tag on it and "poof," like magic… that bouquet suddenly is worth a lot more!

Or maybe Shakira is clenching one of those roses between her teeth while she belly-dances her way to the bank… now how much would you pay? Place it up on the shelf alongside those dozen roses, and because of its branding and celebrity sponsorship, you're paying a ton for a bunch of cheap crap. Don't be that person. Ah, the brutal truth of sexy marketing. That, ladies and gents, is the mean streets of every beauty counter or drugstore aisle. What is a person to do?! We're about to make you street smart; welcome to "Know Your Ingredients 101."

Tanis' & Neddy's Sidebar: Gone Fishin'

Let's talk about the age-old *"bait and catch"* it never fails. When it comes to cosmetics, or the opposite sex, if it looks good, smells good, or feels good, we are sold. Neddy is a recovering self-proclaimed "pretty packaging" addict, which is not at all uncommon. Having both owned our own spas with a huge selection of retail products, we have witnessed the "look good, smell good, feel good" decision-making process firsthand. The beauty industry knows the bait and by God like all good fish, we are going to bite regardless of the consequences. We may want to return the stuff later due to breakouts, a busted budget or just lackluster results, but to resist nibbling on what's dangling off that delicious little hook is damn near impossible.

This is exactly what companies are counting on to make a profit, which we want them to do, of course, lest they go out of business. But when that margin is too steep for the lack of quality active ingredients, then it turns into a straight up rip off. Sit back and watch. Fishing can be a spectator sport!

Case in point: in our spas, we do our due diligence to have myriad options with a range covering most skin conditions and most budgets. We do our research to make sure we carry brands that are in line with our ingredient standards. However, some companies have invested more in brand marketing and packaging than others. 99% of the time when clients are browsing our shelves, they're immediately drawn to products with the fancier packaging, and rarely ask if the contents are as fabulous as the appearance. A "blind trust" comes over them, ironically based on how the box looks. We found ourselves having to advocate for less attractive brands when we felt they would have a better result for the client. It seems funny having to persuade them to choose the "Plain Jane" product housed in a simple white jar with a sticker label and at half the price knowing that it would actually help their skin condition *better* than a "Fancy Pants" product in slick packaging. In fact, some products had the same active ingredients at equal or higher potency than "Fancy Pants", but the struggle to get them to buy the "Plain Jane" product was real. And then forget it if "Fancy Pants" smelled like strawberries and cream and felt like the velveteen rabbit; it was impossible to pry the jar from their hands. These "look good, smell good, feel good" lures can cause the consumer to pay double if not triple for a product that often contains a lot of fluffy filler. Why are we such suckers? We're leaving that to our shrinks. More importantly, why the price gap?

It costs money to keep you taking the bait. From the gold embossed bottles to the retail real estate in department stores or big-box retailers, to celebrity endorsements. It all has a price tag. Usually, a huge percent of the price tag has nothing to do with what is actually in the container. What you are paying for is all the "extra touches" after products have left the production line. Details retailers and consumers ultimately demand. Ah… the fresh scent of capitalism. But like mama always said: "the devil's in those details". Or, at least in this case, the extra expense is in those details…so buyers beware.

Even though the lure of sexy products is still alive and well, there is a revolution, of sorts, occurring in the industry right now. Consumers are actually growing tired of being duped! Well, you don't say! People are demanding more "clean" products, content transparency, less fluff, and more sustainable ingredients and practices. Think of this chapter as our ode to enlightenment. That, or a slap in the face while screaming "WAKE UP SISTA!" At least, it is better than the twelve-step program Tanis had to enroll Neddy in for "pretty packaging" liberation. Read on and set yourself free.

Remember that ingredients are listed
from the highest quantity to the least.

The first line is the tell all to what you're really getting, which means it's no surprise when many products are made up of inexpensive fillers. Is the first ingredient water? How much are you willing to pay for that?

Next, know your fillers. In skin care and cosmetics, a filler is a component in the formula used to create bulk, texture, or lubrication. It helps make that primer feel extra silky, but it is not an active ingredient, nor does it always improve the performance of the product. Most fillers are harmless, but there are others that are sketchy. Some are humectants attracting water to the epidermis either from deeper within the surface or from humidity within the atmosphere. Moisture is locked in the epidermis, thus improving hydration. Still other fillers are surfactants; responsible for breaking down fats and oils acting like skin detergents. And others, well, they're just taking up space.

Here are some gentle fillers, the "baby's breath" of our bouquet:

• **Glycerin** Also called glycerol or glycerine, is a commonly used humectant in skin care products. Glycerin is in all natural lipids (fats), whether animal or vegetable although modern-day skincare products have gravitated to synthetically manufactured versions. Synthetic glycerin is relatively inexpensive to manufacture, and it yields a consistent result. Glycerin not only replenishes but also restores the skin. This is because it is one of the many substances found naturally on the surface of our epidermis, making it a great ingredient to support our own natural moisture barrier, maintaining and defending the skin's overall health.

There has been some concern about whether using products with glycerin will pull too much water from deep within the skin when there isn't enough humidity in the air for it to lock onto. We should note that any humectant in pure form can escalate water loss in lower layers of the skin into the epidermis when the climate is without moisture. It is because of this that humectants are usually used in lower concentrations and combined with other emollients or oils to prevent transepidermal water loss (TEWL).

• **Water/Aqua** It's pretty self-explanatory. It won't hurt your skin, but it won't change it either. And it's cheap.

• **Aloe** Also popular in skincare products, aloe is known for its many benefits including its antibacterial, soothing, healing and anti-inflammatory effects. Aloe's cooling gel consistency and non-greasy hydration make it popular in products for oily skin.

However, this ingredient has recently been getting into some hot water in the beauty industry. Aloe comes in various forms, both naturally and in products. You may see it on the label as decolorized aloe, aloe latex, or aloe water, the sap-like gel that comes straight from the leaf. According to Prop 65, which is a regularly updated California state law that keeps you in the know on ingredients linked to cancer, aloe is noted on the list. However, only "non-decolorized, whole leaf-extract" which basically is the liquid portion of the aloe vera leaf itself was linked to cancer in rats when ingested. That being said, the alarming aloe that is on the list is not applicable to your skincare products. Also, the ingredient has been on the list for two years and there has been no evidence that aloe applied to the skin can be detrimental. "Aloe vera is a safe ingredient to use in skin products," says cosmetic chemist Perry Romanowski. "But this is a good reminder that just because an ingredient is natural, does not mean that it is automatically safe and effective."

Which leads us to the things in our bouquet that may be a little thorny:

• **Propylene Glycol** Propylene glycol is a small organic alcohol molecule used in products as a skin conditioning agent and penetrator. However, it is also classified as a skin irritant, commonly associated with causing dermatitis and hives in humans. Get this! Propylene glycol concentrations as low as 2% were found to manifest eczematous sensitization effects on the skin [54].

• **Sodium Lauryl Sulfate** Don't you just love those "Scrubbing Bubbles" commercials with those cute little guys racing around your toilet taking all the hard work out of cleaning your latrine? Adorable! We know. So, it's natural when you think of "cleaning" you think of "foaming bubbles". Sodium lauryl sulfate (SLS) is the ingredient used in most products that froth, as it is an inexpensive and very effective foaming agent. However, it is also what the FDA uses as an irritant on test subjects so that they can try out other products' ability to soothe the irritation! So just think what SLS is doing to your pretty peepers as it dribbles over your face in the shower when you rinse that very bubbly shampoo from your hair. Better get the Visine® that stuff gets the red out.

In 2000, a *heavily altered* article from the Journal of the American College of Toxicology was posted to the Internet. The paper was modified to make false claims that SLS caused cancer. This rumor was debunked by Snopes.com and there is no scientific evidence that links the use of SLS to cancer. Now there's some *real* Fake News. Nonetheless, SLS does have properties that break down the skin's moisture barrier, stripping it of its naturally occurring sebum, which is still bad news.

• **Petroleum and Mineral Oil** We remember when petroleum jelly (Vaseline®) and mineral oil (Hello Ponds® cold cream!) lived in our grandparents' medicine cabinet… alongside the castor oil and rubbing alcohol. What the hell is mineral oil, anyway? And why is it a filler to steer clear from? Mineral oil is a petrochemical derivative. It comes from that black gooey stuff that made the Beverly Hillbillies able to live in Beverly Hills. Oil, that is, black gold, Texas tea. And if you're wondering if it's the same stuff that makes your car run, that wouldn't be entirely untrue.

Mineral oil is actually not a mineral at all. Instead, it's a semisolid mixture of hydrocarbons known as white petrolatum which is derived from petroleum. To produce gasoline, petroleum must go through a distillation process. Mineral oil is the colorless, odorless liquid byproduct of this distillation process. It's a highly refined product and is used to make petroleum jelly and paraffin wax and often ends up in cosmetics. During the distillation process, many other substances are isolated, and the more crude products include automotive fluid, kerosene and asphalt. These are known to be a human carcinogens based on evidence from studies in humans as reported by The National Toxicology Program in their Report on Carcinogens. [55] Another important consideration is the concern that mineral oil could be contaminated with toxins linked to an increased risk of cancer. Scientists state that cosmetics might be a relevant source of the contamination [56].

Now that you know where it comes from, let us explain why we think it's a "no-no" for your skin. Our rationale is plain and simple: mineral oil does not provide nourishment, nor is it beneficial for your skin. Simple as that. Since it is occlusive, it just hangs out on top of your skin, smothering you, like your aunt, at Thanksgiving dinner. Some might argue that it is moisturizing. True, but that is only because it is sitting on top of your skin, preventing moisture from escaping. Whoop-de-doo. With tons of alternative ingredients on the market these days that actually penetrate, nourish and provide correct hydration to your skin, why be a dinosaur? It's time to step into the modern era folks.

For an amazing alternative to these petro-chemicals, check out **Keys® Avo Gel**. It's the closest thing we've found to Vaseline® ever; from our friend the avocado. Keys® also makes some great personal lube called **PurPlay** and we love the fact they acknowledge that sex lubes of the past have been made by men for men and that "PurPlay is designed for women... and for men... but mainly for women!" That makes us laugh and feel happy. You can find their healthy, slippery solutions at www.keys-soap.com.

Now that we've filled you in on fillers, there is another term you must have in your toolbox, because unfortunately, many product fillers can be comedogenic.

Comedogenic means: tending
to cause blackheads by blocking
the pores of the skin.

Now why would anybody want to go and do that? Beats the hell out of us. Imagine suffocating. Yep, that's what is happening to your poor, defenseless pores when you coat your skin with thick, stifling, and heavy creams or cosmetics that contain comedogenic fillers. Now, you don't want to be a featured guest on Dr. Pimple Popper's YouTube channel, do you? We thought not. Although popping zits keeps us employed full time and Neddy openly admits to having "fun" this is not so much fun for you. Contrary to what some people believe, your skin does not suck up everything you layer on it. Remember, skin is like our armor, it sure would be a crappy one if it didn't serve its purpose! That being said, many ingredients found in products just camp out on the surface of our skin. In theory, skincare products are designed as a treatment to improve the overall appearance of the epidermis. Yet some ingredients either do absolutely nothing or more damage than good; such as comedogenic fillers.

There is no precise way to test for comedogenicity, but the rabbit ear test has been the go-to method for years. Rabbit ears were discovered to be more sensitive than human skin and they reacted swiftly to comedogenic ingredients. Cosmetic rabbit ear testing was done by patch testing ingredients on the inner ear of rabbits; reactions were analyzed both visually and microscopically after a few weeks. A list of comedogenic ingredients was created including 12 categories: lanolins, fatty acids, alcohols and sugars, waxes, thickeners, oils, pigments, silicones, sterols, vitamins and herbs, preservatives and "other ingredients". Testing results then ranked components from grade 0 to grade 5, with 5 being the most comedogenic [57].

Nowadays, animal testing is taboo, so some studies are conducted on human specimens. Nice! For a solid list of common clogging compounds, go check out the journal article about comedogenicity at: https://bit.ly/2Tbj8zC. Then go look at your labels, you may be surprised. When shopping, look for products that say non-comedogenic, and you'll already be a step ahead.

Your skin will let you know what it likes and what it doesn't. Your skin doesn't care about the price, the brand name, or the celebrity, so neither should you! The best thing you can do is to know your skin type, skin condition, and the active ingredients in your products. Be aware of what works. The standard ingredients that have been shown to be active in skin care products are the following:

- **Tretinoin (Retin-A®)** A vitamin A derivative that works by helping the skin exfoliate rapidly. It also rebuilds the skin's tissue. It's commonly used for anti-aging and acne annihilation. In the USA, you need a prescription. In Mexico, you do not. Just sayin'.

- **Vitamin C (Ascorbic Acid)** A potent antioxidant that can neutralize and remove oxidants, such as those found in environmental pollutants and after exposure to ultraviolet radiation. Helps to inhibit melanin production, while increasing collagen. Commonly used in the treatment of hyperpigmentation and in anti-aging products.

- **Vitamin E** An important fat-soluble antioxidant that protects the skin from various deleterious effects due to radiation by acting as a free-radical scavenger. Features anti-inflammatory and wound healing properties. Commonly used for anti-aging, hyperpigmentation, keratosis, psoriasis, wound healing and dermatitis.

- **Niacinamide** A topical vitamin B_3 (niacin) that has anti- itch, antimicrobial, vasoactive, photo-protective, oil regulating, and lightening effects depending on its concentration.

Improves elasticity and is commonly used for anti-aging and hyperpigmentation.

- **Hyaluronic Acid** A key molecule involved in skin moisture. Can be sourced from plants or animals. Improves skin elasticity, hydration, texture, and structure. Commonly used for anti-aging and hydration.

- **Alpha Hydroxy Acids** A group of organic carboxylic chemicals that can be naturally occurring or synthetic. Benefits include: exfoliation, hydration and brightening.

- **Salicylic Acid** A beta-hydroxy acid with anti-inflammatory and exfoliating benefits. Commonly used in the treatment of acne and psoriasis.

These are effective active molecules, and what you should search for on ingredient lists. If a product has multiple active components, expect the price to creep up. After you conduct your label analyses and you find a product that you are interested in, you then need to ask yourself if you can commit to spending that amount of money on a regular basis. Can you commit and stick with the program? Because it is common knowledge in the skincare industry that products have to be used continually to see change over time. So, sit down and have a heart to heart with your bank account and your inner disciplinarian. Remember, product frogs never blossom into barefaced beauties!

With all the competition in the industry, there is always a new trendy ingredient that is the answer to all your skin sins! Whether it's a magic meteorite (yes, it's trending), a celebrity endorsed melon, or just straight up make believe, it's sure to deliver skin bliss... yeah, right. Investigate them to find out if these "groundbreaking" ingredients really work. We know a couple of gals at www.asktheestheticians.com who will live chat with you and help. Sure, most companies will boast about their clinical results, validating the effectiveness of their products, but don't swallow the hype too fast. It is pretty easy for companies to conduct private clinical tests to get the "percentage results" they need. Studies should be double-blind, placebo controlled and hopefully with results published in a peer-reviewed journal article (which is where almost every reference in this book comes from).

This also applies to more affordable products, you know, the stuff that lives on the big box retail shelves. Read the label. Does it contain ANY standard active ingredients? If so, where on the list is the active ingredient? (Hint, except for some strong acids, if it's not within the first five components listed, it ain't doin' a darn thing!) Or is it just a fluffy filler placebo that feels good, smells good and has some cute packaging?

Here's our strategy for finding the perfect product. Have a clear vision of your overall skin goals. Know your skin type and condition. Identify the ingredients that can help your skin get to where you want it to be. Then, sit down and be honest about your budget. How much are you willing to spend on your skincare regimen? Can you afford to buy and replace these products regularly? Start with products that are at a price point that you feel good about, include the actives you are looking for to attain your specific goals and are non-comedogenic. If it works, that's great! If not, step up the price point and try again. Let your skin be the guide; it will pretty much tell you if something is working or not. Sound overwhelming? That's why God made estheticians and why you are smart enough to have one. They should be able to walk you through the process, honor your budget and sell you active products and exchange the ones that are not working for you. If not, find a new one; not a product esthetician. And let this be your new cautionary motto: "Buy Blind. It's Pimple Time!"

WHAT YOUR ESTHETICIAN **REALLY** WANTED TO TELL YOU

- "Buy Cheap. Break Out," although a fun title to our chapter, is not always accurate. There is no strong correlation between product quality and price in the beauty industry. Know your budget, read your ingredient lists and get help.

- Fillers are cheap and add bulk, texture, or lubrication to products. Most are harmless, some are horrific. Know the difference and decide how much you will pay for fluff.

- Look for non-comedogenic products and stop suffocating your skin.

- Are there active ingredients in your products? If not, they're not doing shit. Choose the ones that will help you achieve your skin care goals. Professional products sold by estheticians and doctors usually have high levels of active ingredients. Ask and you shall receive.

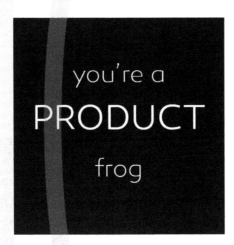

you're a
PRODUCT
frog

10

YOU'RE A PRODUCT FROG

STOP HOPPING

Bless you child, for you have sinned and spent more than most people's annual income on beauty. The global median per capita household income in 2013 was $2,920, according to Gallup metrics [58]. The cosmetic industry is bringing in about 62 billion annually in the US alone. And the American Society of Plastic Surgeons report Americans spent more than $16 billion on cosmetic plastic surgeries and minimally invasive procedures in 2016, (the most the US has ever spent on such operations) and... you get the picture.

As two self-proclaimed product junkies, we kind of get this. But by all means, please let us share with you what, we don't get.

Tanis' Client Case #2,590:

CLIENT PROFILE: First time client, Caucasian, female, 34 y.o., Fitzpatrick rating: III, skin condition: jacked up (meaning all over very superficial breakouts with pustules and comedones not indicative of hormonal or food induced acne).

Client: Can I ask some questions about the product I am using?

I noticed one of the brands is one that you use in your shop.

Tanis: Of course.

Client: Well, I started using the X moisturizer because my friends said it was so awesome and it smelled just like coconuts, so I dropped $60 and bought it online.

Tanis: Say what?? You mean the moisturizer that my brother lubes up his nipples with to prevent chafing before he runs 26 f*cking miles? That moisturizer is *way* too heavy for you and is probably causing this breakout. And when you buy on-line, 1) you have no expert advice from an esthetician who would most likely recommend something that is at least a good match for your skin, 2) you have no idea how old the product is and the older it gets, the higher the bacteria, yeast and mold content (this is no bueno), and 3) let me guess, no refunds.

Client: Well, true that. So, I gave it to my friend. And then I was reading this organic beauty blogger's post and she recommended everyone should buy Y moisturizer because it is so ab fab!

Tanis (interjects): So, I bet you went online, dropped another $60 and bought the Y moisturizer that is so ab fab... for my desert rat grandma who tans with a foil reflector six months out of the year, that is.

Client: Yeahhhhhhh….so, I'm thinking it might be breaking me out so…

Tanis: …you bought it online so you gave it to your friend?

Client: Yeah. So, like, then I was at this really ritzy resort spa and my mom was getting a facial and I got a massage.

Tanis (thinks): Smart lady to choose the massage. It's an estie in-clique secret that high end resort spas are where estheticians go to get experience when they are green and basically have no clue. It's like the new helicopter pilots that fly the tours over the Grand Canyon to get their hours, you know, the ones that always crash.

Client: The esthetician comes out to the lobby, glances at my skin (covered with 5 layers of MAC) and proclaims that I really need Z moisturizer to clear up my skin because it's so broken out.

Tanis: *sighs* You mean the one designed for 15-year-old boys with testosterone induced chronic grade IV acne? You mean that one?

Client: Like, yeah, so... another $60 and they didn't have a return policy so…

Tanis: I wish I was your friend.

Be the Yin of the Nike tag-line Yang and "Just Stop It". Just Stop It. Stop It!

Neddy's Client Case #814:

CLIENT PROFILE: First time client, Hispanic, female, 64 y.o., Fitzpatrick rating: IV, skin condition: minimally wrinkled with moderate hyperpigmentation.

Client: Please help me with my skin! I have spent hundreds of dollars trying to get rid of these wrinkles and brown spots and nothing is working!

Neddy: I'm sure you have not tried everything! What *have* you tried?

Client: Well, first I used that product by that movie star, you know, the one on the TV...

Neddy: ...infomercial?

Client: Yes. And I spent a couple hundred dollars, and she said it would brighten my face and get rid of my wrinkles and look!

Neddy: Ok. How long did you use it?

Client: Two whole weeks! Most days. Well, I guess about 12 days total.

Neddy: Let me explain. Like all of us, you have been working on those wrinkles and brown spots your entire life; in your case, 64 years. Both go down to the dermal layer and when skin is affected that deep, it takes time and consistent use of any product, even the best product, to make a difference.

Then the story repeats and repeats with the product as the only changing player. Some skincare lines this client used were great, with just the right ingredients for her skin. The issue was that she did not *consistently* use her products. We will see an improvement in fine lines and hyperpigmentation, under the best of circumstances in about 3-6 months meaning:

1) The product has active ingredients matched with the user's skin type and goals.

2) Application is twice a day every day.

3) You are practicing sun protection.

Don't be the fickle frog: do not hop and change lily pads for the sake of changing. Unless it's a licensed esthetician getting intimate with your bare-naked face under an illuminated magnifying lamp, we would be extremely slow at taking anyone's recommendations. We don't care how many followers they have on IG or how drop dead gorgeous, and famous, and skinny, and rich (ok, we digress) they are. A reputable shop has: a skin professional, quality products that deliver results, plus a healthy return policy, oh, and an esthetician who knows how to use a mag lamp. We are so confident in our recommendations to our clients we will take anything back that is not making their skin BETTER than when they came in. We don't have to worry about losing our shirts with this policy because, well; we are trained professionals. And shirts are overrated.

Tanis Says It's Easy: be like a scientist. Hell, if I can be one you can, too. Have a professional analyze your skin and discuss your goals. Choose the top two goals you want to focus on; if you are breaking out, that's number one. After they assist you in determining products that will help you achieve those goals, possibly after trying samples for a minimum of three days, choose one or two products. During the initial trial, if your skin experiences any negatives, depending on the reaction and severity, immediately discontinue use, then take the appropriate steps (call 911 in the event of an allergic reaction, we are not kidding here). Otherwise, call your doctor, but at least call your esthetician.

We recommend you do not start on more than two new products at a time. If something changes for the worse, the elimination game is going to be easier. Even if it is a comprehensive line that has five or six components, we still recommend starting a few at a time, using them for at least two weeks, and then adding on the others. We have learned this the hard way. If you are using a quality product, your other goals may get simultaneously addressed. If not, use the same method to address them. Use the products as recommended! Yes, that means washing your face and getting them on even when you come dragging in late, very late, from Coachella, your little sister's bachelorette party or for us mature ladies, our book club. Stick with them and be consistent. If they are improving your skin, not worsening it; use them passionately with great fervor for 3-6 months. I repeat, twice a day, every day, for 3-6 months. Take before and after pictures, we know you have a selfie stick.

Neddy Says Hold Up: listen, we are not cold-hearted "Higher than Thou" estheticians. We're human, and we are women, too! Trust me when I say it's hard! I have seen Tanis put her hands up to shield her eyes as she runs through the cosmetic section of department stores, drugstores, and even the duty-free shops at the airport. I have fallen down that rabbit hole a time or two, as well.

It's a slippery slope – and at the
bottom is a pile of unused cream
ready to fill up your nearest landfill
and empty your bank account.

The media is shoving new trends down our throats daily by young, hot, vixens. The pressure to look flawless is real. But let us "get real"; no one is walking around in a Valencia IG filter or digitally enhanced with FaceTune. So, don't be too hard on yourself.

When you jump from product to product, trend to trend, seeking an instant fix and then not getting that instant fix, you're only causing more stress, which can cause more breakouts! And when that "miracle product" works no miracles on you, worry sets in, which is an open invitation for unwanted wrinkles.

Here's the deal, you have to *know* your skin, *listen* to what it's telling you and remember your esthetician is your skin therapist. When you're in touch with your protective armor and what it needs, you won't be easily sold. Yeah, I said SOLD. Because that's what the media, Hollywood, and advertisements are doing, selling "the dream" in the form of a cream. They either use the strategy of saying your sexiness will improve tenfold, or use fear tactics that tell you you're damned and doomed and will live a life of ugliness, loneliness, and despair without their product. I love this saying: "No one can drive you crazy, unless you give them the keys." Don't fall victim to pressure, take your time with your products, and give them some opportunity to work. It can be difficult because as women we are very aware of our physical appearance and we zero in on our "flaws" with precision. Then we feed our insatiable insecurities with the newest trend. Respect your skin enough to do your due diligence. Your fountain of youth or miracle remedy may be collecting dust in your medicine cabinet all because you didn't have enough patience and discipline to see it through. Remember, it's YOUR skin, and what works for others may not work for you. I can assure you you'll get your groove back the minute you take control of your skincare and stop letting it take control of you.

WHAT YOUR ESTHETICIAN **REALLY** WANTED TO TELL YOU

- Stop It.

- Stick to your skin care regimen decided on by you and your esthetician. Was Rome built in one day? Neither is a Roman Goddess.

- It's your life and your skin: *you* choose what's trending.

- Send all the money you are going to save by following our advice to "The Keep It Clean Campaign" to buy much needed cleansers for women in the Los Angeles Downtown Women's Center.

PART II

WHY IS MY FACE COVERED WITH BROWN PATCHES?

*"In a dark place we find ourselves,
and a little more knowledge lights our way."*

~ YODA

Hyperpigmentation is the numero uno complaint of ladies with melanin-rich skin. It also presents in fair females, males of every ethnicity and basically anyone who is not living under a rock literally. Usually harmless, skin discoloration can be emotionally distressing and some even find themselves avoiding social situations, especially if they involve activities typically done bare-faced. We never want you to have to check in with the local dermis report to see if the forecast brings clear complexions before attending a beach party, hiking, logrolling, or anything that tickles your pickle.

Our Take: People want fast results and by God, as an esthetician, if you don't deliver, you may get dumped. We have seen facials that promise immediate elimination of hyperpigmentation. Really? Just like cellulite, it kind of makes you wonder why anyone has either if there is an easy fix. We know we look at our plump posteriors every day and think exactly that. Don't be duped! Your esthetician probably isn't telling you that combating uneven skin tone will take tenacity and money… and it still won't happen overnight. Why the discoloration dodge?

Are they lazy? Your esthetician should be giving you many recommendations after learning about *your* preferences for erasing brown patches. This takes research and research takes effort and time. Then, your journey should be carefully monitored. How much exfoliation can your skin actually handle daily? Are the products working? Does the plan need to be modified? Is your esthetician being a good guide? Or is your face interfering with their social media life? This is going to take knowledge and energy from both of you to form a winning team and beat hyperpigmentation. Don't pick a lazy teammate.

Are they clueless? There are certain gold standard ingredients that, like eggs in the 80s, got a bad rap. And like eggs, the benefits versus the concerns need to be discussed. Maybe they haven't taken the time to investigate these ingredients, are unaware of alternatives and, most importantly, don't know which ones actually work. Hands-on experience treating discoloration is important, and firsthand experience treating their own face is priceless. Ignorance is not bliss; you need an estie with some hours doc'd in their logbook.

Are they greedy? Your estie may not be telling you about all the strategies to manage your melanocytes because some of the best ingredients are only offered through a doctor's office. And your doctor may be unaware and/or uninterested in the new natural alternatives to the traditional prescriptions that are being offered at organic spas. Pay attention, you will be married to these products for at least three months for optimum results. Choose how you want to spend your money, or they will choose for you; not always in accordance with your desires, comfort level, and budget.

Are they scared? Has your esthetician ever informed you, you have hyperpigmentation? Whether it is obvious or currently invisible to the naked eye, they should let you know they know. And then, they should frankly ask you, "do you care"? Like a stain on your favorite blue dress, sometimes you just don't want to wash away a memory. If this describes you and your relationship with your melasma, and it has become a comfortable part of your appearance, they should respect that decision. If you are ready to pummel the patches, they should rise to the challenge. Either way, they shouldn't be afraid to ask.

If you find yourself relating more and more to Lady Macbeth, take heart and know there are ways to lighten up and even completely eliminate hyperpigmentation. We break down the main triggers of skin discoloration and then present a multitudinous amount of ingredients and products that can help. We agree with the Lady and are here as part of your team. Our mantra? Well, "Out, Out Damned Spot," of course. We've pulled out the stops and presented different pathways for you to ponder on your own journey to complexion perfection. And when you find that cellulite treatment that *really* works, give us a shout out... we are sure you will.

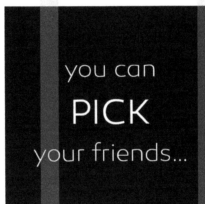

you can
PICK
your friends...

11

YOU CAN PICK YOUR FRIENDS…

WEAR YOUR GENES

And you can pick your nose… wait, different lesson. The chalk talk here is that you can't self-determine your genetic ethnicity. In other words, you were born to two other humans and your DNA, which dictates a lot about your coloring you inherited from them. We are born with different amounts of melanin and even slightly different <u>types</u> of this potentially problematic pigment, which leads to varying vulnerabilities for different ethnicities; darkly pigmented persons are the most at risk of dyspigmentation [53]. And along with our skin tone, we also inherit whether (and to what degree) the triggers for hyperpigmentation will affect our skin. You can't pick your family, but you can control what your skin is exposed to and if you do develop hyperpigmentation, you can choose whether to relinquish or kick it in the ass.

Melasma, chloasma, freckles, hyperpigmentation, sun spots, brown blotches, whatever you may call it, is a mystery, as the exact etiology, or cause, is unknown. So, a little skin physiology, please… melanocytes are pigment cells in the outermost layer of the skin and they provide our skin with color. Melanocytes produce melanin in varying degrees based on the level of an enzyme called tyrosinase; the more tyrosinase, the darker your skin will become. Tyrosinase is triggered by ultraviolet

(UV) exposure, skin trauma, and hormones. Sun exposure (with a hereditary predisposition) is the strongest predictor on whether you will hyperpigment [59][60]. Now that we know the three main triggers: sun, skin trauma and hormones, let's talk about the three primary ways excess melanin presents itself.

The Sun Trigger: Hyperpigmentation is a term used when there is too much pigment in the skin. It is usually scattered over the face and is a common description for what is often seen in Caucasian, sun-damaged, aging skin. The role of the melanin is to protect the nucleus of the cell from damage and that's why melanin production can go ape shit crazy on us; it's being produced to protect the DNA of the cell from getting damaged by UV radiation! Hence, the deep, dark tan that looks so sleek and sexy is actually screaming deep, dark, damage! A specific type of melanin called eumelanin creates dark skin tone; the more eumelanin your body produces, the darker your skin will be. Fair people, like, say, the Swiss or Irish have a small production of melanin, while ethnically Asian people produce a slightly different type of melanin called pheomelanin. Nonetheless, sun exposure influences when the melanocytes become activated and produce more melanin, making the skin become darker in appearance. Sometimes with freckled, speckled outcomes.

The Skin Trauma Trigger: PIH or post-inflammatory hyperpigmentation is a term used when skin turns dark because it was damaged, becomes inflamed, and then attempts to heal. Again, a study shows that the darker the skin, the more prone it is to experience PIH with dyschromia being the second most common diagnosis among African Americans, but failed to make it into the top 10 most common diagnoses for Caucasian patients [61]. We often see PIH after someone has performed an unprofessional pimple popping, especially if they scratched a whole chunk of tissue off during the process (another reason to get regular facials). PIH can also occur from conditions like eczema or psoriasis. Our clients ask us how long their post pimple popping pigment is going to persist? The best-case scenario is weeks, worst-case scenario, years or eternity. Which leads to the next most common question, how the hell do I get rid of it?

Tanis' & Neddy's Sidebar: American Pickers

In the antique business, the term "picker" refers to individuals who spend their time digging through other people's attics, barns, and garages looking for particular items; shall we say, valuable vintage items, that can be sold to an antique specialty store or an online collector. You might have even seen the reality TV show. And if you're reading this, Mike Wolfe, IG us if you find some cool vintage chick jackets, preferably corduroy circa 1970. But if you hear "picker" at an esthetician convention or in the break room of your local day spa, the word takes on a whole new meaning. In the skin biz, "picker" is used to describe someone who is suffering from Dermatillomania aka Excoriation Disorder (ED). ED is a mental disorder related to obsessive-compulsive disorder and is characterized by picking, not through someone else's shed, but picking at one's own skin. People may pick at healthy skin or irregularities that they feel or see such as pimples, skin tags or lesions (that they themselves have made from picking). It usually starts at puberty, but can begin in children as young as 10 or in adults, 30-45 years of age [62]. About 1.4% of Americans experience ED, and more women are affected than men [63]. Now, we all have those occasional moments when we just can't stop scratching at a zit! You know the ones that give up a little pus and blood but you still feel that plug hiding below the surface and dammit, if you have to jab it with a needle you are going to get that bugger outta there. But with ED, the picking is chronic and uncontrollable. The American Psychiatric Association says that the following signs and symptoms will be present in a person diagnosed with Excoriation Disorder [64]:

- Recurrent skin picking resulting in lesions.
- Repeated failed attempts to stop picking.

- The behavior causes distress and the avoidance of social situations, like going to the gym or beach.
- Symptoms are not caused by a substance or a medical or dermatological condition.
- The symptoms do not more accurately describe another disorder.

So why the sidebar? It is not uncommon for people with ED to seek out estheticians who will help them "extract" and heal their skin. When we have seen them as clients, they have nothing to extract since they've already removed any type of blemish from the skin along with a substantial piece of flesh, leaving a large lesion usually with post-inflammatory hyperpigmentation. An esthetician can offer some topical healing agents, but what we really want is for anyone experiencing ED to seek support. There are medications and/or cognitive-behavioral therapies that can greatly reduce symptoms. We strongly encourage you to get help, or help someone you know to get help, if you believe ED is affecting a life. Contact The TLC Foundation at www.bfrb.org and also see a dermatologist for the best strategy to encourage healing and avoid scarring. And pick up a copy of "Skin Picking, the Freedom to Finally Stop" by Annette Pasternak, Ph.D [65]. We care about you, how you feel, how you look, and how you feel about how you look. It matters. You matter. Set yourself free.

The Hormone Trigger: Melasma is a term used when the pigment is clumped in larger patches, appearing as a "moustache" on the upper lip or as a "butterfly" on the upper cheeks and the sides of the forehead. Melasma is recognized to be more common among women than men and more common among Latinas, Blacks, and Asians than among Whites [59]. And certain ethnicities are more prone to melasma, a common skin condition characterized by irregular light brown to dark brown patches on the face [53][59]. Melasma is the form of hyperpigmentation that is associated with hormone fluctuations caused by pregnancy (chloasma), menopause, oral contraceptives, or hormone replacement therapy and will often disappear when the hormone imbalance corrects itself (such as after giving birth or going off of the pill). An estimated 50% to 70% of pregnant women in the US develop melasma [66]. Estimates of prevalence among pregnant Latina women are between 50% and 80%, and one third continue to have melasma for the rest of their lives [60]. A recent study reported that 8.8% of Latinas [67] and 40% of Southeast Asian women living in the US have melasma. Although not instigated by UV exposure, it will worsen with sun exposure. The combination of UV radiation and hormone-related melanocyte stimulation will not only worsen the condition, but may allow the melasma lesions to remain visible for prolonged periods of time, potentially forever. And not only does sun exposure make it worse, but heat can also exacerbate the condition, making it very difficult for those melanocytes to keep their cool. Saunas, working out at the gym and even a hot steamy kitchen can trigger melasma… honey, it might be time to order take-out.

No matter what you call it, having uneven skin tone from patches of excess melanin is a leading complaint among our clients. We also know that having brown blotches can cause emotional distress and pose a negative impact on the health-related quality of life. It can be downright heart wrenching to work with clients who so desperately want even skin tone and who struggle to understand what is happening and how to make it stop. Don't lose heart. There are proven ways to create even color in skin and we are here to present different options to you. Then, you have to do your part, begin a treatment regimen and stick to it with all your guns.

WHAT YOUR ESTHETICIAN **REALLY** WANTED TO TELL YOU

- Hyperpigmentation is caused by "hyper" melanocytes triggered by the sun, skin trauma and hormones.

- You were born with specific genes that dictate your genetic predisposition to hyperpigmentation, but that doesn't mean you can't defend yourself from it and obliterate it.

- You wouldn't have sex without wrapping up the winkie, would you? Do the same when you go outside and practice "Safe Sun" by enveloping your skin in sunscreen. They don't call 'em "sun spots" for nothin'.

- Stop picking and get an esthetician... who has a mag lamp.

LOCATION

LOCATION

LOCATION

12

LOCATION, LOCATION, LOCATION

IT ACTUALLY IS ABOUT YOUR HOOD

Knowing the three main triggers of hyperpigmentation, we can immediately eliminate losing sleep over one of them, our genetics. There is not much we can do about our genetic predisposition. The hormone predicament, however, *can* be manipulated… to some degree. If you are with child, or trying to NOT be with child, we get it. But the choice to use hormones is very complex and personal and hyperpigmentation is just one consideration. And what your hormones do on their own can go back to the genetic thing. So, what's left? You see what's coming here folks… put on your thinking caps and solve the piece of the pigment puzzle that's possible. Drum roll please… as Tanis' mama often shouts, "Get out of the sun, you know you're not supposed to be in the sun. What are you doing in the sun? You know what the doctor said about the sun…" etc. etc. etc. And mama was right.

Do not overlook and do not underestimate the importance of photo-protection. If you are not going to at least try to block your ass from the sun, don't even bother reading the next section or buying products to help with hyperpigmentation. Just march your salami skin butt right into the tanning salon and tell hyperpigmentation, tell melanoma, tell all the wrinkles and spots and f*cked up skin problems caused by the sun to "come on and bring it! Hit me with your best shot… fire away!" And then, live with the aftermath. But if you are not quite ready to cry craven, keep reading.

Depending on where and how you live, you are going to have to use more or less sun protection. We mean realistically; we're not going to tell our gaming buddies who never leave their parents' basement or our friends in Denmark to slather on the SPF 50 come October. Your location is a consideration. Other than that, let's consider some UV protection options:

- Stay indoors, especially between 10am and 2pm (not very much fun, but effective).

- Stay in the shade (almost not as much fun and possibly not very effective).

- Wear sun protective clothing such as that made by **Solumbra**® cute clothes and umbrellas, but it's difficult to stay 100% covered, especially when it's hotter than hell outside. Our most favorite items are the water clothes made for snorkeling, don't go to Hawaii without them! (Fashionable and effective).

- Wear sunscreen. (Practical and effective).

- Become a vampire. (This could possibly be the most fun and effective, not based on actual experience).

Sunscreen comes in a variety of forms, such as creams, sprays and even powders. They also contain different active chemicals. Here's the breakdown, but first, we're calling a sidebar.

Tanis' & Neddy's Sidebar: Chemical Free

All matter is made of chemicals. Then what is matter? To simply answer this question, we will state what is NOT matter. Energy is not matter. We recognize energy in a variety of forms such as light, heat, gravity, sound. You get the picture. If you believe you've got one, your spirit or soul is probably not matter. Basically, everything else is matter. If it occupies space and has mass, it's matter. If you can see it, smell it, touch it, taste it, breathe it… it is matter. A chocolate éclair? Matter. Sperm? Matter. Air molecules are made up of very small atoms that occupy space and have mass, matter. Carrots? Matter. Facial lotion made from organic carrots? Matter.

You're doing great! A+. Now, let's recall lesson #1, all matter is made of chemicals. Chocolate éclair… chemicals. Sperm… chemicals. Air… chemicals. Carrots… chemicals. Facial lotion made with organic carrots… chemicals! Yes! Say it OUT LOUD! We don't give a damn if you're on a Virgin Atlantic flight in upper class sitting next to Kate Hudson, say it right now, shout it! "My organic carrot facial lotion is made of chemicals!" Kate will appreciate your righteousness.

Embrace the word "chemical." Better yet, learn to love it. We are all composed of wondrous and amazing chemicals and without them, we would only be heavenly bodies drifting through the ethers praying we had some f*cking chemicals to get this party started. Look, it's ok – don't cry. We have been brainwashed, more precisely green-washed, by the "natural" beauty industry into thinking that the word chemical is a dirty word. That clean, pure, organic beauty products that come from Mother Nature are "chemical free" and those are the only products that smart and environmentally hip people would ever dare bring into their homes. Stop sounding like a blockhead. We Googled this shit, and we were supposed to learn about matter in the fourth grade. Now grow up, learn some science, and for goodness' sake, never again let the words "chemical free" pass in succession from your mouth. Never. And if they accidentally do, please do not be holding this book when it happens. Thank you.

A-ha! Now you understand why we had to have that sidebar. For some dumb reason (well, it's actually a smart and tricky marketing strategy), sunscreens that only contain active mineral ingredient such as zinc oxide and titanium dioxide that reflect UV radiation are often referred to as "chemical free"! WTF?! Well, now that we have all been educated about the stupidity of those two words used in succession which we will never mention again, we will use the term "physical sunscreen" to refer to products that only contain zinc oxide and titanium dioxide that physically block the sun's rays, and "sunscreen" to refer to the lotions, sprays and powders that contain other active ingredients besides or in addition to zinc oxide and titanium dioxide.

When choosing sun protection, there is new data constantly being released, so we would be fools to make conclusive statements about much of it. But we know some things for certain and we encourage you to decide upon which sunscreens are best for you and your family based on:

1) Efficacy

2) Safety for you

3) Safety for the environment

4) Whether you would actually wear it

Let's ponder protection so you can pick your perfect product! Early civilizations used local plant products to protect their skin from sun damage. Ancient Greeks used olive oil, Egyptians used extracts of rice, jasmine, and lupine plants and some Polynesians even to this day slather on coconut oil to soothe sunny skin. A paste made from zinc oxide has been used for thousands of years to block rays. But with skin cancer being the numero uno "big C" in the US, the highly researched, advanced sun protection

1) **Efficacy** Sun protection products guard us from ultraviolet type A (UVA) and ultraviolet type B (UVB). UVA are the invisible rays that penetrate deep into the dermis, the skin's thickest layer. Unprotected exposure can lead to premature skin aging and wrinkling (photoaging),

and suppression of the immune system. That's why your herpes may flare after you've been out catching some rays. UVB rays will usually burn the superficial layers of your skin. It also plays a key role in the development of skin cancer. UVA and UVB both suck, so you will want to ensure the product you choose is "broad spectrum" and protects you from both.

The sun protection factor (SPF rating, introduced in 1974) is a measure of the fraction of sunburn-producing UVB rays that reach the skin.

SPF 15 means that 1/15th of the
burning radiation will reach the skin.

Now this, of course, is assuming the sunscreen is being applied thick and evenly (at a dosage no less than 2 milligrams per square centimeter (mg/cm^2). Whaa? Trust us, that is one copious amount of product. Don't have a metric ruler lying around at the beach? We don't either, so get that shit on. Make a friend, perhaps one you would want to date, and ask them to help you apply it to your back, that weird space on the side of your rib cage, perhaps that bald spot on your head, perhaps not; you've got this.

Even and heavy application is the reason spray and powder forms of sun protection are a little hit and miss, pun intended. They'll work if a puff of wind does not blow them away onto your beach blanket buddy and you actually get it on thick and strong. Good luck.

Is higher SPF always better? In 2011, the FDA proposed to cap SPF values at 50, calling any rating above that "inherently misleading" [68]. Our friends in Canada, Europe, Australia and Japan agree; they've capped their products at SPF 50 [69].

Some studies even show that if there is a higher number on the label, people may believe they are fully protected and stay out in the harsh sun even longer [70]. Also, be forewarned, a higher SPF does not last or remain on the skin any longer than a lower SPF and you've got to re-apply as directed, especially when you are dancing the salsa in Miami in August or swimming... anywhere... in any month.

There is little evidence that
sunscreens with SPFs higher than 50
provide additional health benefits.

In the USA, we even had to be wary of words on the label until recently. New labeling and testing standards proposed by the FDA over 30 years ago got stuck in perpetual purgatory until June 2012. Finally, they approved new measures to help consumers decipher how a product works, if it is water resistant and to what "type of water" (sweating versus swimming) and the prescribed application of at least every two hours. Our sunscreens have to include "Drug Facts" but they are looser than the regulatory agency in Europe, the EU. For example, we do not have a regulation deeming it necessary to mention whether the contents contain nanoparticles of mineral ingredients, but the EU does. More on nanoparticles in a minute.

The most important part of sun protection is to not give a damn and just get it on. Neddy once dared Tanis to use straight up zinc oxide (you know the white stuff in a metal tube found in the diaper rash section of the drugstore) all over her face when they were at the beach. The picture may still be on Instagram. Be fearless, our pallor peers, the ones judging you on your sunscreen application will not be the ones paying for your skin cancer medical bills. Screw them and save your skin. And if our memories serve us correctly, Huey Lewis and the News once sang "It's hip to be pale".

2) **Safety for You** Now that you know all sun protection is made of chemicals (good for you smarty pants!), do any of them actually contain ingredients that may be harmful? Yes. The FDA approves 16 active ingredients for sunscreens; two of them are the minerals zinc oxide and titanium dioxide. And some are powerful free radical generators,

estrogenic, mutagenic, and may even cause skin cancer. Damn. And then there are nanoparticles, more on that in a minute.

We could write a book about the FDA's shortcomings and successes (mainly shortcomings) regarding regulating sunscreen and, more importantly, how they are (or are not) approving new ones, but this is not that book. We encourage you to keep up with the latest research because, by the time this is published, things will have changed. Currently, the EU has approved four new ingredients that are stuck in FDA limbo. They are superior at protecting the skin from UVA more than ingredients approved in the USA.

So, if you happen to be in St. Tropez and need sunscreen, you may consider: Tinosorb S, Tinosorb M, Mexoryl SX and Mexoryl XL. Here's why, British researcher Brian Diffey evaluated the UV protection of four US and four European sunscreens, each of which had an SPF value of 50 or 50+. On average, he found that the US sunscreens allowed three times more UVA rays to get to the skin than the European products, which included these modern UVA filters [71]. Because our choices are probably limited to US ingredients, here are some "questionable" ones to investigate:

- Micronized zinc oxide (nanoparticles, read about it in "Safety for the Environment")

- Micronized titanium dioxide (nanoparticles, read about it in "Safety for the Environment")

- Oxybenzone (banned in Hawaii, read about it in "Safety for the Environment")

- Octinoxate (banned in Hawaii, read about it in "Safety for the Environment")

- Octocrylene (strong allergen and potential free radical generator, may damage DNA)

- Vitamin A (best to avoid sunscreens with this ingredient… keep reading)

Our last sunscreen tip has to do with antioxidants. You know how we love us some good vitamin A, C, and E. They are antioxidants, which "quench" or reduce the negative impact of free radicals caused by UVA.

So, it makes sense to mix a magical
elixir of sunscreen and antioxidants
such as vitamins A, C and E – right?
Wrong!

Those vitamins are not very stable and when you put them in a cream, that's hanging out from year to year in the bottom of your beach bag, cooking on a black sand beach in Hawaii, and then exposed to some crazy rays, you can bet that those molecules are having a breakdown, sometimes forming harmful byproducts [72]. For example, a technical report issued by the National Toxicology Program indicates that vitamin A additives common in sunscreen, such as retinoic acid and retinyl palmitate, may speed up the development of tumors and lesions on sun-exposed skin [73]! Welcome to the wacky world of science and esthetics, but have no fear, your esties are here! Save your money and your skin and keep the antioxidants in your food and night cream. Amen.

3) **Safety for the Environment** Okay already, it's time to talk about nanoparticles. Sounds like something we could be flying our Jedi Starfighter through. Nano? Non-nano? Nano Nano? Okay Mork, nanoparticles are so small they have to be measured in nanometers. 50,000 nanoparticles could fit within the width of a human hair! Recently, companies have micronized or reduced the size of zinc oxide and titanium dioxide down to nano-size, which was first a blessing, then a curse. See, the very small size actually allows the easy application

of these minerals to the skin without the wearer looking like a mime or Geisha. And even though we prefer Geishas over mimes, no one wants to show up to their local coffee house looking like they're ready to do a fan dance. Contrary to urban legend and some self-proclaimed yet extremely popular "beauty experts", these micronized minerals probably do *not* get absorbed into the skin (74)(75)(76)

But the problem is this, if you are using spray or powder sun protection with micronized zinc oxide and titanium dioxide, you can snort them right up your nose. This goes back to the "safety for you" topic since we do not know a whole lot about inhaling or ingesting (think kids licking their hands or triathletes licking their sweaty upper lips) these micronized molecules. Philip Moos and colleagues conducted experiments with cell cultures of colon cells to compare the effects of zinc oxide nanoparticles to conventional zinc oxide powder. They found the nanoparticles were twice as toxic to the cells as the larger particles. The concentration of nanoparticles that was toxic to the colon cells was equivalent to eating 2 grams of sunscreen about 0.1 ounce [77]. And inhaled titanium dioxide particles have been linked to lung tumor development [78]. 'Nuf said. To make things more tricky, labels do not have to tell you whether the particles have been micronized. This makes it challenging to avoid nanoparticles and stick with the larger sized stuff that is safer.

Then, there is the environment. A study conducted at the University of Toledo showed that titanium dioxide nanoparticles can mess up the functioning of microorganisms in our water supply. When we jump into a river, ocean, or shower to get off sunscreen, the particles wash off and harm the bacteria that actually help water to stay clean and in ecological homeostasis [79]. But wait, there's more. Titanium dioxide and zinc oxide nanoparticles produce significant amounts of hydrogen peroxide when exposed to UV, and that creates stress on marine phytoplankton. The study was conducted on a real Mediterranean beach full of tourists covered with sunscreen [80]! The tourists had a grand time; the phytoplankton, which are the basis for the oceanic food chain and feed coral and fish (which then feed larger fish, humans and sea mammals like dolphins) all while producing oxygen, did not.

The ingredients oxybenzone and
octinoxate may damage coral reefs.

And coral pulls the nasty greenhouse gas, carbon dioxide out of the air. Life on earth depends on the survival of coral and if we keep killing it at the current rate, scientists predict that by 2030, over 50% of the world's coral reefs may be destroyed.

But in 2018, Hawaii was the first state to pass a bill written by David Inge, the Governor of Hawaii, banning these two potential coral killers. The ban was described by state Senator Mike Gabbard as "a first-in-the-world law". Expect to see about 70% of sunscreens pulled from the market by 2021 to comply with Governor Ige's bill. The Miami Herald announced in 2019 that by a 6-1 vote, the Key West City Commission banned the sale in the city limits of sunscreens that contain the ingredients oxybenzone and octinoxate. Some "experts", particularly those working for the sunscreen companies, have surmised that the reef damage is being caused by global warming. We agree. But why ignore one possible cause of coral corruption based on another? Let's face it! Global warming is difficult to control and the choice of a sunscreen is not. So Key West has decided to do everything possible to decrease the stress on their precious reef system. The ban will go into effect on January 1, 2021.

4) **Will You Wear It?** If you won't put it on, for whatever reason: texture, opaqueness, smell, glide, it won't protect your skin, so don't even bother buying it. Start by reading the ingredient list. If it has stuff in it you don't want, set it down and walk away. Don't even bother sampling it on your skin because you know how your senses can take over in a flash. We don't care if it's pink and smells like a piña colada, use your brain and not your nose. If it has the ingredients you are down with, give it a go. Follow the directions, too. Some sun creams call for application to damp skin and others must be spread on dry dermis. And then once you have all this figured out, wear it!

Also check your foundation for an SPF rating, especially if it's a liquid. If it has an SPF of 15 and that is enough protection for that day's activities, there is no reason to put on another layer of sunscreen that is also SPF 15. In this case, 15 + 15 does *not* equal 30! We love products that do double, triple or even quadruple duty. If it moisturizes, has an SPF, has a splash of color to even skin tone, and contains active ingredients (for example, ones that calm down melanocytes to prevent hyperpigmentation), all the better! Sometimes, less is more.

WHAT YOUR ESTHETICIAN **REALLY** WANTED TO TELL YOU

- Protect yourself from the sun. Creams with high SPF are best. Avoid powders and sprays, especially with mineral nanoparticles and oxybenzone and octinoxate that do harm to the environment. Avoid octocrylene and keep your vitamin A in your food and night cream, but leave it out of your sunscreen.

- Sun protection is the key to the puzzle of hyperpigmentation. You need to use it to help unlock even skin tone.

- Look for SPF products that are multi-functional and can also moisturize, even skin tone and deliver active ingredients.

- And in the words of Marvin Gaye, "Let's get it on."

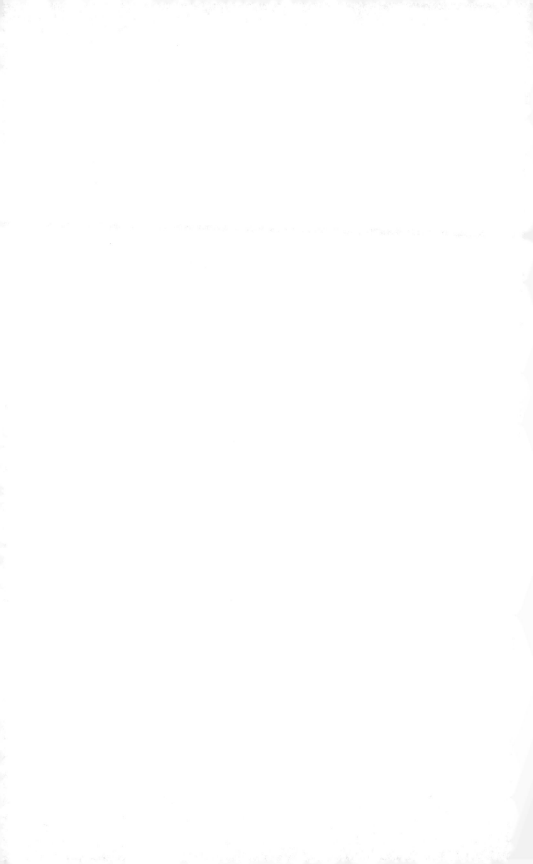

look on the
BRIGHT
side

13

LOOK ON THE BRIGHT SIDE

HYPERPIGMENTATION IS NOT FOREVER

When it comes to eliminating hyperpigmentation, there's more than one way to shine that penny. When you combine all the hundreds of ingredients and thousands of products that can do just that, we figure there might be just about a zillion ways to zap it. But we'll keep it as simple as possible and reveal the three easy steps you need to take to get the job done and a variety of ingredients to choose from for each step.

Here are the three steps for erasing hyperpigmentation:

1) **Exfoliate:** out with the old cells, in with the new.

2) **Calm:** chillax your melanocytes.

3) **Protect:** shield from the sun.

Here's the clincher. You must commit your time and invest your money and unwaveringly stick to the program; twice a day, every day, for at least three months to see results. Some people say it is easier to accomplish this during the less sunny months, but we say there is *never* a good time to do what you are about to do. If you are wholly and entirely ready to banish your hyperpigmentation forever and ever amen, then buck it up sister, and let's get started. In the words of the great Jedi Master, Yoda, "Patience you must have, my young Padawan."

Step 1: Exfoliate

Some Classic Ways to Exfoliate Skin:

Vitamin A Exfoliation is critical. You need to remove the old over-pigmented cells to achieve even skin tone. That's where the vitamin A comes in. Vitamin A derivatives used on the skin are known as retinoids (and are not recommended during pregnancy). So, how do they work? Retinoids irritate the skin, causing it to make new cells more quickly. We're sure you've seen a house makeover show on HGTV with a remodel. Think of it like that. First, you've got to do the demo. Tear down the old to get ready for the new. Down comes all the old, hyperpigmented, photo-damaged jacked-up cells. Then in comes the construction crew. Reinforcements are installed, more collagen, elastin and other architectural components to hold up the new and repairing tissue. Your fresh skin is installed on top of the reinforced support structures. It has less damage and discoloration than your old facial facade and soon you will enjoy your newly renovated face! But not all retinoids are created equal. Let's break it down.

• Retin-A®, Renova®, Avage® and Tazorac® are brand names for tretinoin, for which you need a prescription. Tretinoin is also referred to as retinoic acid. What's missing here? Ah, a blast of trumpets sounding from heaven as the clouds part and the Saint of Anti-Aging swoops down and hands us the holy grail of youth elixirs, the ark of the covenant of creams, and as it was in the beginning, so shall your skin be in the end. Amen. This shit WORKS! This one ingredient will do all the things that every anti-aging product promises, but few actually deliver. Wrinkles? Check. Sagging skin? Check. Photo-aging? Check.

Age Spots? Check. Acne? Check. Pre-cancerous skin cells? Hell yeah! Check. Somebody stop us! An extra 30 layers of dead skin cells hanging around? Check, check, and check! This stuff is your best bet for quickly exfoliating your skin while eradicating hyperpigmentation. And all those other benefits? Just think of them as Bonus Time.

Although tretinoin is wondrous for many skin types, keep in mind people with darker skin may have increased sensitivity to this ingredient. In a 40-week, randomized, double-blind study conducted with 54 patients who had skin of color to determine the safety and efficacy of 0.1% tretinoin in the treatment of post-inflammatory hyperpigmentation (PIH), tretinoin was effective, however, 50% of patients experienced retinoid dermatitis (skin irritation).

If Retin-A® is so miraculous, why isn't everyone using it? A slow ramp up is required for the successful onboarding of retinoic acid. Using a pea sized dollop every three to four nights for about six weeks will help the skin slowly begin the "tear down" and then go into repair mode. After, patients can use it every two to three nights. This approach helps limit the redness and peeling that occurs [81]. Skin may look worse during this initial phase, but by week 24, most people's skin has dramatically improved. Slow and steady wins the race. Also, you'll want to avoid using retinoic acid if you are pregnant, breastfeeding, or have rosacea. Its use may also have to be limited if using it with vitamin C or acids. Have a thorough discussion with your doctor about what to expect before filling that prescription; and, as always, use common sense.

• Retinol and retinyl palmitate are also vitamin A derivatives, but they must first be converted by special enzymes into the active metabolite retinoic acid to have any effect on skin cells. The problem is the conversion rate is low and varies greatly among individuals. Also, these forms are more susceptible to breaking down when exposed to air, rendering some products useless before they even hit your skin. Yes, retinol products promise to be gentler on the skin than retinoic acid and that is because they are less biologically active! Gentler, but far less effective (if at all) than retinoic acid. Decisions, decisions...

• Vitamin A propionate is the newest addition to the Royal Family of vitamin A. The TL; DR version goes something like this: Goldilocks walks into a spa and an esthetician presents her with some vitamin A acetate. Goldilocks declares, "This molecule is too small." Then the estie pulls out some retinyl palmitate and Goldi balks. "This molecule is too big." Then the estie gets her act together, goes to the skin convention and spends eight hours perusing the aisles, slathering cream on every square inch of her exposed body before falling asleep for 20 minutes in an LED bed and polishing off her day by getting liquored up with her colleagues at Shenanigan's Irish Pub and having to take an Uber home *before* showing Little Miss Blondie her skin convention score: a dropper vial full of **VivantSkinCare**® vitamin A propionate to which Goldi screams, "Now this is the shit I was looking for because this molecule is *just* right" and runs off into the woods with the bottle. Dr. Fulton, the scientist who co-invented Retin-A®, also patented this middle weight molecule that delivers a mean punch. It was designed to result in the least amount of irritation while providing the greatest amount of efficacy to consistently clear and control acne and reverse the signs of photoaging. And to do so more than any other non-prescriptive retinoid. Tretinoin is still the Queen, but vitamin A propionate seems to be the next in line to the throne.

Some Alternative Ways to Exfoliate Skin:

We still recommend using prescription strength retinoic acid or vitamin A propionate for the exfoliation step of this pigmentation plan for previously mentioned reasons. Alternatives would be to use retinol (which may or may not work) with a physical exfoliant such as a scrub or microdermabrasion. If you feel that retinoic acid is challenging to use for any length of time or perhaps you are pregnant or breastfeeding and want ingredients on the "safe for everyone" list, then the following info is for you. We understand the desire to have even toned skin while using products and ingredients that you love and feel comfortable using. Therefore, we are going to share a few other ways to lighten up. Just keep in mind that consistency and patience will be paramount when using these alternatives.

Alpha hydroxy acids, such as glycolic and lactic, help to slough off dead cells. An esthetician can apply a strong peel or a weaker formulation can be used as often as daily. If you have small localized patches of pigment (like an age spot), your doctor may choose to freeze them off (cryotherapy). It is as effective as a laser treatment, more reliable, cheap and less likely to cause side effects. Hear! Hear! Pregnant? You've got this. Use a scrub and products with a retinol alternative such as **Eminence® Bamboo Firming Fluid**, **Neroli Age Corrective Eye Serum**, and **Coconut Age Corrective Moisturizer,** aloha!

Step 2: Calm

The Classic Way to Calm Melanocytes:

Hydroquinone acts as the "melanocyte calmer" encouraging new cells not to overproduce the pigment, so you don't keep making more melanin-infused cells as you exfoliate the pre- existing ones. 4% hydroquinone (prescription strength) used with 0.05% tretinoin (and 0.01% fluocinolone acetonide to reduce inflammation) led to complete or near-complete clearing of melasma in eight weeks in clinical trials[66]. Sounds like a dream cream, right? But this skin lightener has its dark side, too.

Hydroquinone has been shown to cause ochronosis, a bluish-black darkening of tissue. Ochronosis showed up most frequently when a high dose hydroquinone (6%-8%) was used for a prolonged period by people with dark skin. In a study conducted in South Africa, the prevalence of ochronosis among skin lightening users was 69% [82].

Studies conducted on rats with high doses of hydroquinone led to unfortunate results, non-cancerous growths when taken orally and chromosomal abnormalities when injected. But take heart, dear readers, all drugs used by us can become toxic as opposed to healing when taken in too high of a dose and/or in the wrong delivery method. And since we are not lab rats tainting our afternoon tea or shooting up with hydroquinone, we eagerly anticipate other studies about human exposure to low doses of topical hydroquinone; the way we actually use it. Dr. David J. Goldberg, a clinical professor of dermatology at the Mount Sinai School of Medicine, reports, "Over 100 scientific articles confirm it is a safe topical for humans; no independent studies prove the opposite."

Then why the ban on products containing higher than 1% hydroquinone in some countries? It seems like a few factors were considered, including increased ochronosis and high levels of mercury! Say what?! Yes, mercury is often found side by side in skin whitening creams because it also does a good job of preventing melanin production and it is very cheap. It's also very poisonous and acute or chronic exposure to it can result in kidney, neurologic, and dermal toxicity [83]. In Saudi Arabia, 45% of the skin lightening creams tested contained mercury above the FDA limit[84]! Needless to say, these results were startling, and a global movement took off to educate people about scanning their creams for this poisonous metal.

Think that products being peddled in the US couldn't possibly contain toxic mercury? **Think again.**

American scientists went on a spending spree to buy every lightening product they could get their hands on right here in the good 'ol USA. They bought products online and at shops including department stores, ethnic markets and beauty supply stores and nearly 12% of the products showed up with mercury! In addition to the word "mercury" being on the label or any derivative of the word (such as mercuric amidochloride) look for the following as indicators to put the cream down and run away... screaming:

- Calomel

- Cinnabaris

- Hydrargyri oxydum rubrum

- Quicksilver

If you have decided that hydroquinone is the way to go, please consider: 2% can be bought over the counter and 4% is sold as a prescription. If your doc prescribes the 4%, work with that doctor to determine the appropriate products and regimen. If buying over the counter, make damn sure it does not contain mercury. Do not use the product for a prolonged period; if you are using the holy trinity of hydroquinone, retinoic acid, and sunscreen, eight weeks to three months should show considerable improvement. Monitor the research; hopefully we will see additional human studies regarding the safety of this helpful agent in the near future.

Some Alternative Ways to Calm Melanocytes:

Hydroquinone Stand-Ins There are ways to interrupt the production of melanin using different agents other than hydroquinone. Here are some options with the ups and downs of each:

- **Arbutin** Is it Halloween? Because hydroquinone just arrived... in disguise! Welcome, arbutin! Everyone got very excited about this lightening agent until they realized it was hydroquinone with a sugar molecule stuck on its backside, so don't get too excited about arbutin if you are trying to avoid hydroquinone. The sugar cleaves off and the active hydroquinone molecule is released. Arbutin seems to be gentler and cause fewer skin irritations than hydroquinone, probably because of its gradual release. However, it is unknown if the concerns regarding hydroquinone may apply to arbutin as well. There might be an elephant in the spa, and its name is arbutin.

- **GigaWhite®** This is a trademarked compound that includes extracts from Swiss Alpine plants that work through the same mechanism as hydroquinone to shut down excess pigment production. A test revealed that GigaWhite® can reduce excess color by up to 24% in 12 weeks in Asian skin. If you find this mountainous mixture on an ingredient list, keep reading. There may be other lightening agents in there as well.

• **Vitamin C** We could write a book (and maybe we will) about how useful topical vitamin C is to solving so many skin quandaries. It decreases melanin production and even acts on perifollicular pigment [85] that's the extra pigment that can hang out around a hair follicle and presents as little dots all over the skin. In a double-blind study, 16 women with melasma applied a cream containing 5% ascorbic acid (vitamin C) to one side of their face and to the other side a cream containing 4% hydroquinone. Everyone used daily sunscreen. The best subjective improvement was observed on the hydroquinone side with 93% good and excellent results, compared with 62.5% on the ascorbic acid side; however, colorimetric measures showed no statistical differences!

And get this, 11 out of the 16 women had side effects due to the hydroquinone, but only one woman had side effects from the vitamin C [86]! Although hydroquinone performed better, ascorbic acid can play a role in the therapy of melasma with little to no side effects. The downside is that vitamin C is unstable, especially when exposed to air. Look for products that contain at least 5% C and are packaged in an air-pump (that is, ironically, devoid of air). It doesn't hurt if they pair vitamin C with other depigmenting agents such as soy and licorice for better effectiveness [87].

• **Kojic Acid** There's a fungus among us, and it's evening out our skin! Produced by, yes, a mushroom; kojic acid seems to be comparable to hydroquinone in its effectiveness. The problem is that like vitamin C, kojic acid is very unstable and is easily oxidized if exposed to air and can react with other chemicals if exposed to sunlight. To overcome this difficulty, some product manufacturers use kojic acid dipalmitate, a more stable derivative. But here's the funny part, but not haha funny because some companies are taking our money when we don't even know if kojic acid dipalmitate reduces hyperpigmentation! We are waiting for studies that put it head-to-head with kojic acid and/or hydroquinone to gauge its effectiveness. Until then, if this is the only active lightening ingredient in the product, we wouldn't bank on it.

• **Licorice** Not the Red Whipped kind or even the black chewy kind (the best of which comes from Australia BTW) but the extract of *Glycyrrhiza glabra* kind that will make your melanocytes sit down and stop talking. The good stuff comes from the root and there are three main components that may show up in your products. They are glycyrrhizin (you may see it listed as glycyrrhizic acid, glycyrrhetic acid or dipotassium glycyrrhizate), liquirtin and glabridin.

Licorice is an antioxidant that will help reduce puffiness and calm down skin, particularly your pigment producers. All three agents act against acne scarring, melasma, age spots and freckling. Liquirtin helps to disperse pigment as 90 Pakistani patients of Nishtar Hospital experienced. In that study, 4% liquirtin was more effective than both 2% liquirtin and 4% hydroquinone[88]! Glabridin is thought to prevent the skin from darkening in the first place and can be used as hyperpigmentation prevention. And thanks to its anti-irritating character, licorice is far more tolerable than hydroquinone.

• **Acerola Extract** Here's a dietary take on the fight against hyper melanocytes. The acerola cherry (not really a cherry, but a berry and not to be confused with tart cherry) grows in north S. America and Central America and has a high level of vitamin C in addition to a lot of other goodies that do wondrous things in our body. Drinking the juice from the acerola cherry, *Malpighia emarginata* DC., suppresses UVB induced skin pigmentation in a study performed on mice[89] and guinea pigs[90]. The fruit is not transportable, so unless you live in the subtropics and grow your own, you can purchase it in powder or supplement form.

• **DERMAPEP™ W220** Our friends over in Korea have patented a complex that is halting the biochemical pathway of pigment in its tracks. DERMAPEP™ W220 contains methyl undecenoyl dipeptide-16 that blocks production at the source; it acts on the hormone Alpha MSH, which regulates pigment. Because of its action, its manufacturer, Tri-K Industries, Inc. claims that it is more effective than arbutin.

Other Hydroquinone alternatives to keep your eye on are soy, mulberry, Illumiscin™, Melaslow™ Daisy Flower (*Bellis perennis*), Indian Kudzu (*Pureraria tuberosa*) leaf cell extract, and niacinamide. All show promising results and many contain anti-inflammatory properties to boot.

Step 3: Protect

Sunscreen Decreasing your exposure to UV rays is of the highest importance when you have practiced the other two steps of this troika. When you are peeling while simultaneously trying to get your tissue to make new skin cells without excess melanin, it is imperative that you do not expose this process to one of the major triggers of hyperpigmentation, the sun. Seek shade, stay indoors, wait until winter, wear a hat and a sick pair of sunnies to look fabulous and be safeguarded. Wear sunscreen; a key component in the regimen of even-toned skin and the eradication of melasma and all things hyperpigmented.

The cool thing is that many companies combined ingredients so you can have an all-in-one cream! Why put on multiple layers when one will do? A fine example of this is **Eminence® Bright Skin Moisturizer** that contains GigaWhite™, bearberry and licorice to lighten, stone crop (a succulent related to aloe vera) to moisturize, and a sunscreen providing an SPF of 40.

Tanis' & Neddy's Sidebar: Anti-DIY

Retin-A, Hydroquinone, and Sunscreen. This is the gold standard when it comes to obliterating brown spots. Let's just cut to the chase. You can monkey around with a million products containing those three essential agents, but if you want to save your time and money, read on lovelies.

We understand we are the generation of DIY. After all, the information you need to do just about damn near everything is on the internet, right? We think Tanis' dad learned how to fix his weed wacker on YouTube. But there are still certain things that you will want to get professional advice about before buying your products through a licensed dealer.

None of us seem to have a problem making time to visit a MAC° counter or Sephora° store in order for the make-up artists to paint our faces and give us advice on application, hottest trends, etc. We willingly open up our wallets to dish out the dough for the glow. But hell no, we won't make an appointment at a medical clinic when we are experimenting with the pigment of our face. We are just going to follow some beauty blogger's advice and go on eBay to buy up someone else's discarded products all in the name of... what?... saving a buck? Being lazy? Thinking we are just as intelligent as the doctor who has spent a decade studying and tweaking out thousands of people's personal pigmentation programs? Really? This is not the time for DIY.

Specifically, one medical clinic option is Dr. Zein Obagi's program. It crushes hyperpigmentation and includes many more powerful agents than just those three big-hitters, making it highly effective. We have seen significant results in clients who have used his first product line, Obagi°. He sold that company and started **ZO® Skin Health**, a new product line we trust because it has been developed by the great eraser himself.

But whatever you do, go to the doctor's office because you will want an expert to customize the program just for your skin and supply fresh, potent, and prescription products. You will also get the moral support you'll need to get back on track when you feel like quitting... and you will. If you choose this pathway, the trick is to get on the products, hit it hard, and then get off of them as quickly as possible. Your doctor will cheer you on to even-toned skin because they know it is achievable and they care!

Combating hyperpigmentation is also a race against time; the sooner you attack it after it appears, the less work, money and time it will take to delete it. But whatever ingredients you choose to diminish dark spots, be consistent and tenacious, and you will experience a brighter tomorrow!

WHAT YOUR ESTHETICIAN **REALLY** WANTED TO TELL YOU

- There are different products to eliminate hyperpigmentation, but whichever regimen you choose, it needs to 1) Exfoliate, 2) Calm and 3) Protect.

- You didn't make hyperpigmented skin overnight, so don't expect a quick fix. "Nothing in the world can take the place of persistence." ~ Calvin Coolidge

- Playing with pigment is not the time to DIY. Work with a doctor or licensed professional to lighten right.

- There are always new products hitting the hyperpigmentation scene. Make sure your esthetician goes to skin conventions to find the latest and greatest and then do your own research.

PART III

DON'T YOU DARE LOOK YOUR AGE!

"The soul is born old but grows young. That is the comedy of life. And the body is born young and grows old. That is life's tragedy."

~ OSCAR WILDE, A Woman of No Importance

Anti-aging is one of the most difficult topics to tackle and at the same time, one of the top beauty concerns across the board. Unless you're talking to a 20-year-old eagerly awaiting their next birthday, no one that we are aware of looks forward to getting older. It may not be politically correct and it is certainly not fair and far from being evolved and enlightened, but there are enough stats out there that point to the ugly fact that looks matter.

Our Take: Good looking, young, sexy folks make more money, get more promotions, and receive more positive attention from others. Period. Google "Looks Matter Statistics" or "Women Age Discrimination

Statistics." Be forewarned. Not a heart-warming read here, sisters. Just because there are laws against it, doesn't mean it doesn't happen. And to confuse matters, when we say "anti-aging," are we talking about healthy habits to increase the quality and maybe even the quantity of life or are we talking about getting a head-to-toe rebuild by Dr. 90210? In either case, it's time to bust open this timeless taboo and speak up. So why wouldn't your estie?

Are they lazy? Why would I inform you about drinking hyaluronic acid to help alleviate menopausal dryness or taking DHEA to keep collagen levels high if I don't sell it? Why would I tell you about how Botox® works if it takes up my time and I don't even use it? Why would I tell you that exercise is the best way to ward off Mr. Reaper if I don't even do it myself? Why? Because I'm f*cking lazy.

Are they clueless? Most states do not mandate continued education for licensed estheticians, but they should. The beauty industry is a billion dollar one and everyone wants a piece of this pie. One way to do this is to develop new products that actually work! Thousands of new anti-aging options are released each year; just recently we discovered a new vitamin A derivative that may rival Retin-A. Estheticians need to continuously self-educate, conduct research, and then bring their findings back to the treatment room for the ultimate product challenge. If this is not happening, your estie may be a "product *pendeja*."

Are they greedy? There are two major groups of professional beauty institutions: the medical-spas and the more "natural" facial spas. If you are in a medi-spa, topics like Botox®, fillers and face-lifts are the norm, but most individuals in these facilities probably do not offer organic products, extractions, or a good ol' traditional facial because why the hell would you want "safe" and "natural" when for chrissakes you're shooting botulinum toxin into your forehead? If you own an organic facial spa, wouldn't your clients be horrified if you suggested that if they *really* want to get rid of those nasolabial folds, they should go get shot up with some filler or get a facelift, or both, and just be done with it?... or would they? The professionals in these two categories have been slow to cross pollinate out of fear that the other institution is not in line with their approach to anti-aging and probably, that they may lose clients, and therefore money, to the "other side."

Are they scared? Who's going to say out loud that, statistically speaking, growing old makes you invisible and not valuable and then declares you are starting to look old so you best do something about it? Damn straight, we're scared. We are so scared that we are not even telling you what WE are doing behind closed doors to keep our faces from melting into something resembling a pot of Swiss cheese fondue. Throw us a bone. At least we are writing about it.

We acknowledge and respect all of our clients' desires to stop aging in its tracks and it's ok if you want to only use organic petrochemical derivative free products while simultaneously receiving plastic surgery, fat-melting injections and Botox®. It's also not only "ok," but we salute you, if you really don't want to do a damn thing. We support you, will help to educate you about *your* choices and hopefully point you in the right direction to receive all the resources you need to develop your own "aging gracefully" strategy. Remember that bright eyes, a radiant smile, and glowing skin are ageless and always equal "beautiful." And confidence, compassion, and the ability to make others feel great about themselves are what make the journey worth it. Meanwhile, take a gander at the chapters in this section and perhaps you will discover some new "super-ager" secrets that resonate with you. And Happy Birthday!

fillers
FREAKS
& fabulousness

14

FILLERS, FREAKS, AND FABULOUSNESS

BOTOX IS NOT A 4 LETTER WORD, REALLY

Because our skin care businesses are organic product based, we see many clients that want to use safe, plant-based products. But just because they are not interested in loading up their skin with petrochemicals and perfumes does not mean that they will not fight aging with every weapon they can get their hands on, and we support that. We too have more than dabbled with lasers, injectables and have even tangoed with a scalpel or two, and that does not make us any less committed to reducing our skin's daily toxic exposure. Call us hypocrites if you must, but we are estheticians and yes, "esthetics" are the primary driving force behind our actions, our interests, and what we want to share. So, if this chapter is not for you, we get it. But hand it over to your BFF because we know they are most likely getting a little suminsumin done. According to the plastic surgery statistics from the American Society of Plastic Surgeons, 17.5 million procedures (including injectables, chemical peels and surgery) were conducted in the USA in 2017; up 2% from the year before. Let's break it down so you can investigate your options when a cream just won't cut it.

From our experience, most of our clients are confused about the functions of Botox® versus fillers (such as Restylane®) versus the effects of plastic surgery. Many will ask us about a starlet's recent attempts at clutching onto her youthful appearance and gasp at how all that Botox® has made her lips too big and why that filler has stretched the corners of her mouth up to her earlobes and gawk at the facelift that's made her forehead so flat you could project a movie on it. STOP! You have got it ALL WRONG! We are going to help you understand how these different treatments are used to produce fabulous outcomes and what exactly has happened when you see people who are looking a little more freaky than fab. Then you will be in the position to start your own exploration into the wonderful world of cosmetic procedures and discover which ones may be right for you while avoiding turning into a Real Housewife.

Hyaluronic Acid: wear it, inject it, drink it. As a cellular and molecular biologist, Tanis finds hyaluronic acid (HA), aka sodium hyaluronate (the salt of HA that is smaller and able to penetrate the epidermis) and hyaluronan, a very interesting miracle molecule. It is a polymer of disaccharides (two sugars) which are glucuronic acid and glucosamine: you have probably heard of the latter as a supplement for joint lubrication and health. Together along with silicon, they form the ultimate hydrating particle which can hold 1,000 times its weight in water! It's produced in the body naturally and is highest in concentration in the skin, joints, eye sockets, and other tissues where it helps retain water and collagen providing elasticity and flexibility. HA is a key piece of the biological scaffolds upon which new cells are constructed during skin wound repair and is also involved in the inflammatory response. We remember Dr. Murad teaching us when we were in beauty school, "Aging skin is skin that is losing its ability to hold water." When first hearing this statement, one might be inclined to think that the easy remedy to this parched predicament is to simply drink more water. Unfortunately, after the body has reached its natural saturation point, drinking more just means more trips to the potty. BTW, an easy way to determine hydration levels is by the color of your urine; the closer to clear it is, the higher the hydration[91].

We were determined to trick skin into staying as positively plump as possible without moving to the tropics or spending the rest of our lives applying moisturizer in the bottom of a well (watch "Silence of the Lambs" for details on that). Here's our way.

Hyaluronic acid (HA) was first used as an eye lube and now has slipped its way into all kinds of creams to hydrate skin. We consider it a miracle moisturizer because it can address both intrinsic chronoaging (aging caused by father time) and extrinsic photoaging (exposure to sun and other oxidative stressors). Dehydrated tissue due to intrinsic aging is primarily caused by the rapid declination of estrogen and HA (particularly during and post menopause) leading to dryness (including eyeballs so dry you can hardly wedge them open in the morning), loss of elasticity, wrinkling, aches, pains – can you tell at least one of us is talking from personal experience here? And if you happen to be another lovely that is experiencing this dehydration dilemma, you can attest that it seems to happen overnight. One day a bright shiny juicy smooth purple plum and the next, well, you know what happens to old plums, right? You may have heard of or even used bio-identical hormone replacement therapy – this is a way of keeping your estrogen and HA levels raised and therefore what many experience as a more youthful appearance with maintained plumpness and firmness and less sagging and discoloration of the skin. Extrinsic loss of hydration can happen when the skin is exposed to excessive UVB rays, and it becomes inflamed what we recognize as a sunburn. This causes the cells in the dermis to produce less hyaluronan [92] further reducing their ability to retain water and then, just like Dr. Murad said, we have "aging skin."

No matter what the cause of your dehydrated skin, we have some dream creams ripe for the picking. We actually found a study on a specific product that was published in the Journal of Cosmetic Dermatology. Results show that a Swiss product that incorporates five different molecular weights of HA known as **Fillerina**® was "able to provide an improvement in the appearance of chronoaged skin in subjects showing mild-to-moderate clinical signs of ageing skin on the face." Some study participants reported increased cheek volume and fuller lips; two traits associated with young hotties [93]. And low and behold! Neddy recently stumbled across a sample of this with which she quickly anointed herself and proclaimed a la Veruca Salt "I want it NOW!" Of course, it did not make her plump as fast as Violet Beauregarde after the chewing of Wonka's blueberry gum, but presently it has staved off the needle. Take-home message is, get your hands on some Fillerina® or any other product that contains HA and slather away. Tanis' personal favorite is **Eminence® Strawberry Rhubarb Hyaluronic Serum** applied directly after their **Strawberry Rhubarb Hyaluronic Masque.** You'll want to eat it, but remember Violet's fate and keep it on your face.

The most highly researched benefit of HA is its ability to alleviate aching joints. In 2007, the EMA (Europe's equivalent of the FDA) approved Hylan-GF20 as an injectable treatment for ankle and shoulder osteoarthritis pain. It is a major component of cartilage and synovial fluid that bathes the joints with a thick gelatinous liquid, allowing bones to glide and cartilage to act like shock absorbers. When HA levels drop, dryness sets in and so do creaks, degenerative joint disease and pain. The re-introduction of it in the form of a "lube job" buffers bones, provides resistance to wear and tear, and keeps things working smooth. Speaking of smooth, it is also being injected into the dermis to fill out wrinkles (thus its general name in the beauty industry, "filler"). Since it normally exists in our tissue, HA is a safe way to fill in creases such as the laugh lines between our nose and mouth (known as nasolabial folds) and inflate areas of hollowness on cheeks and even puff your pout. Nearly all challenges with the product come from the actual injection itself as the product is compatible with the human body and over injection with too much product can be immediately corrected with the enzyme that breaks down HA known as hyaluronidase. So, what kind of complications are most common? Bruising and swelling and, of course, sometimes it hurts like hell during the injection, but thank goodness these all go away with time. Yes, there are possibilities of other needle blunders and even a chance that your body will have a less than ideal response, and these have been noted in the Journal of Dermatology & Dermatologic Surgery [94]. But the biggest filler faux pas can be avoided by heeding to that age old adage that "less is more". Remember, when Mae West said, "Too much of a good thing can be wonderful", fillers hadn't been invented. This brings us 'round to breach the subject of freakiness and correct our misinformed client we mentioned at the beginning of this chapter that no, it's not Botox® giving that starlet her new "pucker up Donald Duck" look but it is a FILLER! That's right, our beloved hyaluronic acid that is the *actual* fountain of youth being completely abused and misused. We all know that person who, after a few trips to the doctor's office, goes from looking refreshed to looking freakish, dare we say, inhuman, as certain parts of her face swell and bulge and she ends up with a trout pout and mammoth cheekbones rivaling that of Angelina Jolie's as Maleficent.

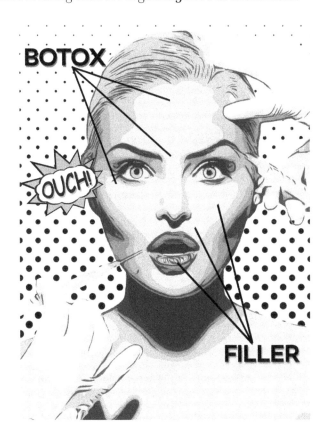

Could this well-meaning but misguided individual of whom we speak possibly be, dare we ask, you? Go take a long look in the mirror, better yet, a deep long gaze into your soul and ask yourself if this is what you meant when you promised yourself at that tender innocent age of 25 that you were going to grow old gracefully. Do you look graceful? We think you do even without all that filler. So, stay fab.

But if you are ready to pull'er into the station and filler'up then we recommend the following considerations. First, here are some brand names to familiarize yourself with, keeping in mind that each brand also makes several products with different densities (we'll get to that in a minute). Restylane®, Juvederm®, and Belotero® are injectable HA products. Stick with FDA approved products, please. We once saw a magazine exposé about some random looney happily charging your cc as she neurotically filled up your face and body with the likes of motor oil, caulk and silicone from Home Depot. We wept when we saw the outcome and boiled over with anger and vengeful feelings for said looney.

This is not the time to shop around for discounts, people. This shit is expensive and highly skilled injectors rightly charge their talents, so if you can't afford the best, stay home. Second, there are FDA approved fillers made with other substances, but we are limiting this discussion to products made with HA. You can research and ask your doctor to see if another product is better suited for the outcome you are trying to achieve. Third, there is a variation in the degree of crosslinking and molecular weight and, therefore, densities of different HA products. The more dense "thicker" products are better for larger areas where you can also get away with more firmness such as the cheeks. These denser varieties also tend to last longer.

Medium dense products are suitable for the nasolabial folds and less dense forms do well in the lip area and under eyes in the "tear troughs." Word up, we have seen quite a few cases of the lumpy bumpies under people's eyes so this is where the art form of injection comes into play, which brings us to our fourth point, you will want to find a highly skilled injector with loads of experience. Do they have a picture portfolio stuffed with amazing before and after pix of actual patients? If you were super awesome at your art, wouldn't you? But they don't? Run. Fifth, keep in mind that some people's bodies burn through fillers much more rapidly than the norm. Tanis happens to be one of those people. Her doctor skillfully injected $3,000 worth of HA into her face, giving her dream cheeks only to be found on the likes of Cher, and sent her off with the lifetime expectancy of 6 months. Three weeks later, she was looking like her cheeks had gone the way of IHOP. "Where did they go?" Her doctor, and she wondered? So once again, her pancake face was syrup'd up and once again, three weeks later, Tanis looked like the pilgrim version of Cher's half-breed and once again poof! Another 3K up in smoke. Metabolism? Acidity levels? Too much damn hyaluronidase?

Who knows? We just hope you don't have the curse of Tanis. Cher, it's still all about you and those gorgeous cheek bones. Sixth, remember that optimistic, wise 25-year-old and be careful... this could be a very slippery slope.

Now here's the fun part most of our clients don't know about and it's relatively cheap and as easy as placing an order on Amazon and doing an add-on to your morning smoothie. Hyaluronic acid is edible! See "Mama's Little Helpers" for the lowdown on the internal lube job.

Botox – It's Not Just for Models Anymore. In 2017, the American Society of Plastic Surgeons reported that 7.2 million sites were injected with botulinum toxin type A right here in the good ol' USA up 2% from the year before. So back to our confounded client. Botox® (or Dysport®) does not give you a protruding pucker or Goliath cheeks (that's filler). But what Botox® does do is stop your forehead from contracting. Here's how it works. Botox and Dysport® are brand names for the botulinum toxin type A. Yes, we are talking about the same group of nasties that belong to the *C. botulinum* family. This is a bacterium that emits a very strong toxin that, when ingested or absorbed through a wound, creates muscle weakness that can lead to difficulty breathing and even death. You were probably warned as a child never to eat food from a bulging can and as an adult never to give honey to an infant, both possible harborers of the bacteria and the toxin. This toxin is NOT what is being used in Botox.

A *modified* and very *specific* and very, very, very *weak* form of this protein is injected into the area of interest, such as the forehead or around the eyes, where muscle contractions are creating wrinkles. Botulinum toxin type A is made in the lab using genetically modified organisms as mini factories for the manufacturing of this modified and attenuated protein yes, we said GMOs. Same goes for many of your meds and those antibiotics that kept your mom alive when she had pneumonia last fall. So, before you go galloping around with your damn picket sign that says "Just Say No to GMOs" be careful what you ask for. Anyway, that's another book. So, let's say your boyfriend washes your new white kundalini yoga outfit with his also new red underpants.

You know that look on your face when you go to tell him he owes you because Fabletics® only makes two styles of workout pants in solid white and he just trashed one of them? That look of imminent trouble results from your angered brain sending a signal to nerve cells which then signal your muscle fibers telling the fibers to contract to convey the crinkled forehead and furrowed brow message of "disdain," but, if you had been treated with Botox within the last four months, there will be no "contraction reaction" because this protein attaches to the muscles in the location where it is injected and the botulinum protein blocks the message from the nerve cells to the muscle telling it to contract. Simply, Botox® is a cell signal blocker.

Word up. Botox® is sold to doctors in a lyophilized (freeze-dried) form. The doctor needs to add saline to it to get it in its liquid form. Tanis was attending a training by Allergan, the manufacturers of Botox®, when the trainer asked the doctors in the room how many of them put in the amount of saline recommended by Allergan. Unfortunately, very few hands in the room went up. That is because these lyin' cheatin' docs admitted to OVER diluting so that they could inject more people with the vial of product. Their unsuspecting patients were getting watered down shots that will not perform as well as the recommended strength. This delivers crappy (if any) anti-wrinkling results. So, if some ad tempts you to buy cheap Botox®, don't plan on it actually working. Enough said. And shame on your integrity-less (new word) docs. That's stealing and for that, you need to go to jail and sit in the 10 Commandments' Corner.

So, Botox® will stop you from furrowing that brow that eventually leads to wrinkles, but unfortunately, it cannot stop your brain from being pissed or can it? Which leads us to this very interesting finding. A grad student at the University of Wisconsin- Madison wanted to test the facial feedback hypothesis that states that a person can alter their mood if they alter their facial expressions. Like smiling (even when you don't feel like it) will eventually lead to happiness and walking around looking mad (even if you feel elated) will probably lead to you feeling pretty cranky by the end of the day. We wonder what happens if we spend the day with our "O" faces on? We digress. Anyway, what he basically did was check people's reactions to situations that could create anger, sadness or surprise, both before and after shooting up their foreheads with Botox®. Well, low and behold, the volunteers did not feel as reactionary to these situations when their forehead couldn't react! Wow! Just think, could Botox® be used to stop road rage? Bar fights? Maybe it should be used in prison to lull the inmates off into frontal lobotomy bliss, all while looking super fly in their orange jumpsuits. Hey, just don't get huffy when we're not surprised at our next surprise birthday parties, just sayin'. You are planning them, right? December and January. Keeping it real.

This goes for around your eyes, too. The little muscles that cause crow's feet can't contract when Botoxed out, which softens your squint lines (BTW this is a GREAT treatment for crow's feet for when a cream won't cut it). Keep in mind that you can still smile, and when you do, your cheeks will push up and will create some little creases. But hey, who's looking at those crinkles when you are beaming your captivating grin?! And as far as "frozen face" goes? Keep in mind that these products can only limit movement in the forehead or tissue on the outer edges of the eyes; everything else remains totally animated, so even though it may be possible to tattoo a crease-free American flag on your noggin, we're thinking that if you can still make faces like Jim Carrey from the eyes down, that you're probably not that frozen after all, let it go.

Collagen – It's Tougher Than You Think. What's all the hallabalooh about collagen, anyway? Collagen is the main structural protein in animals. It is the main component of connective tissue and the most abundant protein in mammals [95]. It's what holds up our face in addition to our neck, knees, butt, boobs, and the underside of our upper arms... you get the picture. Have you ever heard a senior lady declare that one day she just woke up, and she had wrinkles? Can it possibly happen that fast? Yes, when you consider that the levels of collagen in the skin decline at a rapid rate after menopause; approximately 30% is gone after the first five years of not having to buy maxi-pads [21]! Let's break it down before we learn how to build it up.

There are 28 different forms, but over 90% of collagen in the human body is Type I. Collagen is found in skin where it keeps the tissue soft and supple, firm and taut (basically, young). It also exists in tendons, ligaments, cartilage, bone, muscle, blood vessels, the gut (we could go on) and consists of amino acids linked to form peptides which link and fold to form proteins. These proteins wind together to form fibrils, which weave together to form collagen fibers, which may then attach themselves to cell membranes. Many of these steps depend on other factors such as the presence of vitamin C, which makes us think of a hard lesson learned by 18th century English sailors so sit back, sip a Mike's Hard Lemonade® and savor this.

Imagine being recruited to the Royal Navy back in 1747. I know, but try. You board the ship feeling in top form only to be stricken down in a few months to a wobbly waterman. Your gums are bleeding because your frickin' teeth are falling out and your legs are swollen and purple with bruising. You have mates on the ship that are in the same condition as you, or worse, so the crew's Dr. James Lind takes an interest in this swabby sickness. He unknowingly begins the first nutritional, clinical experiment ever conducted and breaks down the crew into six different groups, giving each group a different nutriment; some had cider, others seawater... you get the drift. One group was lucky enough to have been given two oranges and one lemon per day and low and behold, this mess of mariners were miraculously mended! If you haven't guessed by now, these sailors were suffering from the disease known as scurvy and the vitamin C in the citrus cured what ailed them.

The Royal Navy then began making sure that all their sailors had plenty of limes during each voyage, thus preventing this deadly disease while simultaneously giving them the nickname "limeys" and great looking skin! But what the hell does this have to do with collagen? The manufacturing of this complicated protein depends on many nutritional factors, including a vast array of amino acids, enzymes and yes, the critical vitamin C. Without it, the sailors could not produce their 28 forms of collagen and were literally jiggling apart like Jell-O® at a Palm Springs' picnic. Think this is a disease of ancient mariners? The Third

National Health and Nutrition Examination Survey, 1988 to 1994, revealed that 13% of adult males and 9% of adult females in the United States had blood levels of vitamin C indicating scurvy [96]. Ahoy! Hold it together mateys! Someone, grab a mojito and eat your C's or you're not long for the plank! Those limeys could have told you they don't call it Emergen-C® for nothing.

Vitamin C is necessary for a firm face.

You've got that covered, but you probably know that the elasticity of your skin has a lot to do with your genetics, and probably even more to do with your age. But alas, do not throw in the towel so quickly, my fair-haired females (Caucasian women, in general, have lower amounts of collagen and look haggard younger and more often than men and other races). Collagen production can also be affected by lifestyle choices, so let's explore what we can do to keep "up" appearances. First, we want all of our vegetarian/vegan friends to know that collagen is sourced only from animals, so you may want to skip to the next eye-opening chapter of this book if you don't want to harm any critters in your beauty routine.

Second, we need to wrap our heads around the size of this molecule. It's friggin' huge. It is so goliath that a fully formed collagen fiber cannot penetrate the epidermis, we repeat, can NOT sink into skin. Now you may be thinking, "Why the hell am I paying top dollar for collagen infused creams?" Well, we would like to know, too. We also don't want to withhold any info from you either, so we're gonna let you know that there may be some smaller pieces of soluble collagen that can be absorbed, but it is still not possible for these broken fragments to incorporate directly into your intricately woven fabric of elasticity.

Think of it like this: you have a favorite sweater that gets a hole in it: can you fix that hole by throwing a ball of yarn at your sweater? Hell no. Neither can you fix your degrading collagen matrix by slathering on a bunch of collagen cream (this goes for the structural support molecule, elastin, too). There is more benefit to these other three methods of supporting the elasticity of your skin: either inject it, eat it or, better yet, stimulate your own collagen production. Here's how.

Injecting collagen bypasses the big blockade of your skin barrier by using a needle to get this ginormous protein into place. So yes, it is going to provide some support in the area where it was injected, but like all proteins, over time it will break down and you will need to revisit the needle. So, if you've got the time, money, and a high tolerance for pain, we say, "why not"?

Eating collagen which is trending hard enough to make it on the front cover of the "Life & Arts" section of the Wall Street Journal on the very day we were writing this chapter, including such fibrous fortifications as **Collagen BeauTèa®** or **Primal Kitchen's Collagen Fuel®** **Chocolate Drink Mix**. Yum. To find out if these ingested wrinkle stoppers really work, go read "Mama's Little Helpers." Meanwhile, go ahead, have a little collagen with your tea and crumpets.

So that leaves us with the ever so intriguing "stimulate your own collagen in six easy steps." Note the sarcasm. And as the chapter title indicates, getting your collagen levels to increase, or even to get them to stop decreasing, is a little bit tougher but way more beneficial than scoring a jar of St. Ives® Collagen and Elastin Cream at Walgreens®.

1) **Ingest it** Bone broth, gelatin and eggs are some natural sources of collagen.

2) **Eat a healthy whole food diet** Collagen protein is made mainly out of the four amino acids, glycine, proline, hydroxyproline and arginine. By eating healthy sources of protein such as beans, soy, nuts, eggs, salmon and sardines, you can be confident you are capturing the amino acids you need. You'll also need that necessary vitamin C and can glean it from guava, tangerines, yellow bell peppers and dark leafy greens to ensure you've got what it takes for fabulously firm features. You can also pop some supplemental C.

3) **Keep hormone levels high** Are you entering menopause or just over the hill and things are getting a wee bit too much, or uh,

actually too little? Consider bio-identical hormone replacement therapy (HRT) because keeping hormone levels from crashing also means your collagen and elastin (and everything else for that matter) will stay somewhat stable. There is a natural decline in collagen of about 2.1% per year for 20 years post-menopause [21]. HRT reverses this trend and increases skin collagen [97]. There are also drug free ways of keeping hormones high and if you happen to be one of the individuals who doesn't drink, smoke, or eat sugar or processed food, and you exercise and meditate every day, sleep eight hours every night and have a stress-free life, we salute you! Otherwise, have a discussion with a doctor who is extremely experienced with bio-identical hormone replacement therapy and then make an informed and examined decision.

4) **Make an eight-hour date with the Sand Man** Poor sleep equals increased stress hormones, inflammation and decreased human growth hormone (HGH), which you need to stimulate the production of connective tissue and cellular repair.

5) **Exercise** Yup, here it is again. See a trend here people? And again, exercise increases HGH and glutathione… you know how this story ends happily ever after.

6) **Get lit** A study using red light-emitting diode (LED) therapy showed that when measured objectively (that's using scientific tools not your BFF's opinion), there was a significant reduction of wrinkles (maximum: 36%) and an increase in skin elasticity (maximum: 19%) compared to the baseline on faces treated for four weeks. Histologically, a marked increase in the amount of collagen and elastic fibers was observed [98]. Red LEDs also simultaneously decrease the amount of enzyme that tears down collagen praisebetogod!

Our favorite is a wand manufactured right here in the good ol' USA in California by **LightStim**®. This wand is backed by a warranty (you are not going to see this on a device made in Taiwan) and also has a patent on the mixed use of red and infrared light, taking full advantage of all the wavelengths that stimulate the most. What do we see? Improved skin texture, tone and fewer wrinkles. LightStim® also makes a bed of red LEDs, upon which we will spend the proceeds from this book. Thank you, LightStim® for being committed to the firmness of our butts.

WHAT YOUR ESTHETICIAN **REALLY** WANTED TO TELL YOU

- Hyaluronic acid can hold 1,000 times its weight in water. Wear it, inject it and drink it for a plumper, lubricated you. Just don't freakout.

- Botox goes in your forehead and around your eyes to soften or eliminate wrinkles and crow's feet. Find a reputable doctor and look happier and be happier.

- Don't waste your money on collagen cream. If you want to waste money, we've been eyeing this motorcycle/jet ski transformer vehicle that would be way more useful than that cream. Instead, just eat it, inject it or stimulate your own.

- There is a lot you can do to stimulate your own collagen production. Try to incorporate as many strategies as possible, including investing in a LightStim®. If you buy the bed, email us. We'll be right over on our motorcycle/jet ski.

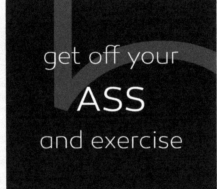

get off your
ASS
and exercise

15

GET OFF YOUR ASS AND EXERCISE

NO EXCUSES

This chapter is about stuff that will save your life, save your face, save your marriage, and save your pocketbook.

Tanis' Take: What if someone could sell you something that would not only extend your life but also increase the quality of your life? That it would make you look younger, decrease breakouts, make your skin firmer, your ass tighter, and increase your overall radiance? Still not interested? But wait... there's more! That it could get you off antidepressants, help you lose extra weight, lift heavy objects and regulate your blood sugar? Still not sold? How's your sex drive lately? Your passion for life? Your blood pressure? Your temperament? Your joy? What an amazing infomercial that would make, right? We would all want this secret pill, book, formula, or whatever the hell this person was selling. Now what if I told you that without it, you may not be around to see your granddaughter's wedding, to take that dream cruise to Alaska or to snorkel on the great barrier reef? Now I'm getting wicked. Is this just for the elite and privileged? Honey child, this time, not only the rich can get the sweet end of the lollipop.

Because this magical elixir, this fountain of youth and euphoria inducing thing is <u>free</u>, you can use it starting <u>now</u>, as <u>much</u> as you want and you will <u>never</u> run out of it! Lord Have Mercy! Praise be to God! Allelujah! We are Saved! Now get up off your ass and EXERCISE! Are you still sitting? Get up and shake it like a Polaroid, jump up and down in ecstatic jubilation, run up and down the aisle of that airplane or mosque or mediation center or wherever you are (because I know you always wanted to do that anyway) and make a lifelong commitment right here right now to move it for the rest of your life! MOVE!!!

Neddy's Take: Really? We work, we raise children, do the chores, cook the meals, some of us have even opted to raise a man of our own (yes, that would be our husbands) so when are we actually going to pack in all this exercise? But then, I saw her just do it. Yes! – Tanis.

Tanis was working a full-time job at a hospital, running her skin care shop and doing 10 (yes, there is a zero after that 1) triathlons per year! When I asked her when she fit in all that training, she used to say "That's why God made 5am." Her HDL is higher than her LDL. Need I say more? She has been my exercise role model ever since and truly walks, well…er…*runs* her talk. And yes, often runs away at the mouth as well, but we still love her. Make an appointment with yourself to exercise and keep it. Value your time and your commitment. We both admit that it takes grit to keep exercise in our routine, but it is actually not an option. Do you have offspring watching? 'nuf said.

With the plethora of information on the internet, exercise science should be common knowledge and perhaps even part of our common sense. But for you, couch potato naysayers, we are about to stupefy you with loads of data. You already know this shit, but we will try to give you as many citations as possible. But we would rather be frolicking in the ocean, or snorkeling the great barrier reef, or skiing in Mammoth, do any of you have a condo there, BTW? We'll bring the face masques and cross-country skis. So here it is… again.

Exercise and its deliriously positive effects:

- **Energy Boost** We know there is clinical data supporting this, but just try it and let us know. Our readers will be our "clinical study". Tell us what you think. Remember, studies have indicated that even low-intensity movement like walks on the beach can increase your vavavoom up to 20%. Survey says: 2 snaps up in a circle on this one.

- **Get Happy** Physically active people have more pleasant feelings than sedentary people. According to a study conducted at Penn University by Conroy and Hyde, they found that not only are movers happier, but the more they move, the happier they are! If you want to feel extra good, go do some moderate to intense exercise, experience the endorphin release, and smile.

- **Chillax** Studies in adults indicate that 30-minutes of aerobic exercise reduces muscle tension by as much as a dose of 400mg of meprobamate, a strong tranquilizer [99]! The relaxation effects were determined by subjective self-reports, through electroencephalogram changes and in the reduction of peripheral deep tendon reflexes. No prescriptions, addictions, or adverse side effects with this "medication".

- **Reduce Tension** Tension reduction induced by exercise lasts for 4 to 6 hours in adults. The mechanism by which physical activity reduces muscle tension is via a central corticospinal effect [100]. An equal reduction of psychosocial stress occurs with both aerobic and anaerobic (like weight lifting) activities [101]. Mainly because it's hard to be competing with your frenemies on Facebook with a badminton racket in your hand. Case reports in adults show that regular physical activity may be helpful in the treatment of panic attacks and phobias [101]. That's why Neddy, always does her jumping jacks *before* going to the rattlesnake round-up.

- **Stay Young** Tanis loves Jack LaLanne. Sidenote, he invented the first breakfast meal replacement shake, a mainstay in our healthy lifestyle. Didn't he look great! No one we know, not even Beto Malfacini, can rock a jumpsuit like Jack. Mr. LaLanne had some serious youth hormones on his side. In one exercise study, HGH, your Human Growth Hormone, aka the Fountain of Youth, increased by 771% after twenty minutes of exercise! High burst interval training works best. There are so many incredible life altering benefits to naturally boosting your HGH, but here are a few of our favorites: increases stamina, lean muscle mass, hair growth, stronger bones and helps regulate fat and sugar metabolism and possibly improves heart function. And coming down the stretch, nose to nose with HGH, glutathione crosses the finish line taking 2nd place! The crowd goes wild! And what is this runner up magical molecule of youth? It is your very own antioxidant made by your body and girl, does it do a body good?! This shit is the key to detoxifying your system (and you thought it was the lemonade cleanse). This antioxidant agent can recycle itself, so theoretically we should never run out, *"should"* being the keyword here. Unfortunately, our modern stressful lifestyle means that most people's glutathione levels are in the toilet. And yes, when our body cannot clean up its act, we are susceptible to disease. Don't be susceptible, be superlative. Just 30 minutes of daily aerobic exercise boosts your glutathione, and your glutes. See you in SoulCycle® and remember, Jack said that the body does not get old from use, but gets old from lack of use. Amen, brother.

- **Toughen Your Skin** And we're not just talking about your keratinized, stratified squamous epithelium. We're talking about your grit, your determination to achieve goals, to withstand a potential TKO and get back up for another round, in essence, to have "tough skin". Dennis Charney of the Icahn School of Medicine at Mount Sinai and Steven Southwick of the Yale School of Medicine spoke to people, including U.S. special forces soldiers and Pakistani earthquake victims, who coped well with a variety of incredibly stressful life experiences. Charney and Southwick identified 10 factors that were found in resilient people that allowed them to be gritty and keep going despite incredibly challenging situations. One of the 10 factors? Being physically fit. BTW, grit has also been identified by Angela Duckworth, the author of "Grit" (our Book Club must read list) as the number one determining factor for success in life [102]. Exercise = Grit = Success. Things that make you go hmmm.... Now, back to your reticular dermis. During strenuous exercise, fibers all over your body, including muscle and tendons, can endure micro-tears, which the body immediately begins to repair. Through your body's effort to repair or replace damaged muscle fibers, satellite cells fuse with the muscle fibers, leading to an increase in muscle fiber cross-sectional area or hypertrophy [103]. In other words, your muscles get beefy! Now, to increase collagen, we are going to go full circle back to HGH. When you exercise, HGH increases and HGH ramps up collagen production. Voilà! Tough skin inside and out!

- **Reduce Disease** researchers aren't entirely sure why, but exercisers have a fortified immune system against future cancers, including breast, and less disease in general. It boosts immunity and helps rid the body of bacteria... could this equate to less acne, too? Estheticians, including us, see that their clients who consistently exercise and sweat have more clear skin.

- **Sweat** This is so *muy importante* we wrote a whole chapter about it. Now go read the chapter "How Dry I Am".

- **Better Sex** Exercise makes us more energetic, more fit, more confident and therefore probably feel more sexy. It can increase arousal and satisfaction for women and decrease erectile dysfunction in men. In one exercise study, the people who had the biggest improvement in physical fitness also had the biggest improvement in their sex life. Strength training can also increase testosterone, the horny hormone. Two birds with one stone? Sexercise! Actually, sex lasts an average of six minutes and burns only 21 calories but sometimes it's the thought that counts! See, we told you this chapter could save your marriage.

- **Live Longer** Oh yeah, that too. About 3.4 more years for 30 minutes of moderate movement five times per week. How shall we spend all that extra time?... hmmm... we know (see previous bullet point).

WHAT YOUR ESTHETICIAN REALLY WANTED TO TELL YOU

- The #1 thing you can do for your appearance is immediately available to you and FREE.

- Compared to a control group that was just told to exercise, another group who planned and scheduled their workouts were 91% more successful at keeping their workout appointments than the control group. Make an appointment, with yourself.

- You are reading this book because you want to know the truth about beauty, right? Would Jack LaLanne have been so hot if he had been a flabby, lethargic, out of breath whiffle-whaffle eating waffles? We thinks not.

- Go rock your jumpsuit. Just do it.

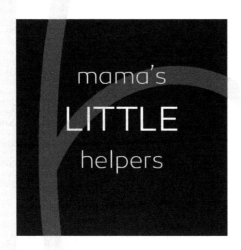

mama's
LITTLE
helpers

16

MAMA'S LITTLE HELPERS

SUPPLEMENTS THAT HELP AND COCKTAILS THAT DON'T

We both remember a time when a caring *abuela* (in Neddy's case) and an elderly kind great-aunt (in Tanis' case) offered us our first shot. No, not standing on a swivel bar stool in Ft. Lauderdale belting out a drunken rendition of "We Are the Champions", but an innocent little spillage from a dusty old bottle of 151 proof Cuban rum (in Neddy's case) and a neat little puddle of green absinthe in the bottom of a water glass (in Tanis' case). We were introduced to these concoctions from our homelands, at the first sign of the common cold or perhaps to ease menstrual cramps but whatever the case, the analgesic and somewhat euphoric effects combined with our young age made for the perfect remedy for what ailed us; sleep.

Flash forward a few decades and we are more confused than ever about alcohol's role in our health routine. To drink or not to drink? Oh, let us give it a few more tries and tell you if we've found the answer to *that* question. Resveratrol is an antioxidant found in grape juice and wine, but we would need to consume gallons to receive a true beneficial effect. Alcohol thins the blood and helps to prevent stroke until too much gives you a stroke and then you've struck out. Isn't the oldest person in the world a vodka swilling 129-year-old German woman? Please help.

The confusion continues and we could spend weeks (more) researching the topic and presenting our data here, but we would miss Hump Day Happy Hour, so let's just sum it up this way. The data actually says what our intuition can tell us. None or very, very, very small quantities of alcohol (like the thimble full that our family first gave to us) seems to be good for you. Please note the first word in the last sentence. For one example of "very little": in Sardinia, Italy (a Blue Zone, one of only five in the world where most people reach 90 years of age or older) many include wine in their daily diet. When Sardinian Zelinda Paglieno turned 102, she was asked her longevity secrets. They included hard work, fresh locally grown food, and "two fingers width of red wine, and no more, at lunchtime every day." Wanna pay for a glass and only drink half? Do you carry a measuring tape around in your purse? Oh, maybe you do. Well, you get the picture.

The way we (meaning the typical person in a social situation) drink is detrimental to our *health* and our *appearance*, especially when we are trying to get the other leg over the top of that chain-link fence sporting our newest pencil skirt and Jimmy Choos. The amount of alcohol consumed on a daily basis thought to be healthy is so low it has made us consider buying boxed, vacuum packed wine that retains its freshness for weeks in order to avoid the temptation of not wasting the bottle. Key word being "consider". But with age, we are getting wiser and more desperate for beauty solutions that work. So, as our age increases, our alcohol consumption decreases and that, we intuitively feel, is a good thing.

As your esthetician, we can usually tell when you've had a little too much the night before your facial. It's your chin. Drinking alcohol inhibits the production of vasopressin, an anti-diuretic hormone. Less vasopressin means more trips to the potty and less hydration for all of your organs, including your skin. The effects are immediate, so you get to wake up to dry eyes, dry mouth, and dry facial skin. Take a hard look at your chin the night after a binge. This is where we can see the most dryness, as the skin can become flaky as soon as the next morning.

Also, when you excessively pee you also lose electrolytes, which can lead to leg cramps and rapid and irregular heartbeat. Have you heard of "sailor's heart"? The term comes from the palpitations that many sea-men experienced after binging on spirits during shore leave. Redness, broken capillaries, exacerbated rosacea and acne, accelerated aging, cancer, and ulcers; the list of alcohol-induced maladies is long. We want you to be on this planet for a long time. So, look fabulous holding that glass of champagne and then you are allowed to pull a quick one by secretly dumping it in the plastic plant in the corner. And when you do imbibe, you can use Zelinda's two finger rule for a unanimous thumbs up!

And what about other vices? The Orchid Recovery and Treatment Center for Women developed a list of the four worst drugs for your face. Now, don't get us wrong, if you are struggling with any of these four or any drug for that matter, the last thing we really give a damn about is your skin. We're concerned about YOU and want you to know there is a group of people at Orchid who can absolutely help you (888.672.4435).

Cocktails That Don't Help:

Methamphetamine aka Meth renders the body unable to repair itself and therefore destroys tissue and blood vessels. It also creates acne, lesions, and accelerated aging. Crystal also causes the salivary glands to dry out, causing tooth decay and even loss of teeth for that ever memorable "meth mouth".

Alcohol Cocktails dehydrate the body, so people who chronically imbibe are usually chronically dehydrated. A friend of a friend essentially "pickled" herself by not drinking water and having a few too many nightcaps every night. Save the pickling for your cucumbers. Long-term drinking can trigger rosacea, a puffy face, a bulbous nose and cellulite.

Heroin Smack causes rapid weight loss, making your skin sag from a loss of healthy fat. Low blood pressure often makes skin and nails have a bluish tint. Opiates cause you to itch, so many junk users pick at their skin, creating open sores. Overall, NOT a glamorous look.

Cocaine Ah the 80's. If you snort it, the loss of the blood to the septum can cause it to erode, endangering your nose to collapse. Sexy. Some blow users feel "bugs" crawling on their skin, which they scratch, forming lesions. You could end up pale, emaciated with a "coke bloat" face. Take Grandmaster Flash's advice, don't do it!

By now you are probably wondering if we actually do, and don't do, everything we are suggesting in this book. Do we really pour perfectly good bubbly on faux foliage? Do we walk the talk? Lead by example? Most of the time, yes, we do. As a matter of fact, the rest of this chapter is specifically based on the contents of Tanis' daily vitamin container (we used hers and not Neddy's because she is so much older and, well, you get the picture). After years and years of research and working with her own medical and naturopathic doctors and being asked by thousands of clients "what do you think about supplements?", the time has come to reveal the list. Read on, consult with your doctor, and welcome to the wonderful and sometimes wacky world of supplementation!

Supplements That Do Help:

Astaxanthin Ever wonder what gives flamingos that adorable pink color? Or shrimp, crabs, lobsters and salmon? It's what they're eating; *Haematococcus pluvialis* to be exact. It is a freshwater green algae that, when exposed to harmful conditions like harsh light, dehydration, or poor nutrition, produces a ton of the carotenoid astaxanthin (which is blood red) to protect itself from UV radiation. When the aforementioned animals eat these algae, they turn pinkish red too. What is so special about this gastronomical goo? It is one of the most fierce antioxidants on the planet. This powerful pigment provides protection and fights off free radicals 6,000 times better than vitamin C, 550 times higher than vitamin E, and 40 times more than beta-carotene, a carotenoid found in carrots and bell peppers (104).

Various benefits for health have been recognized to date, including boosts to the brain [105], heart [106], eyes [107], and kidneys. Other benefits are anti-stress [108], anti-inflammation [109], and of course, enhanced skin health [110] just to name a few.

One human study showed that
there was significant improvement
in the skin when astaxanthin was
applied topically and the participants
also ingested 6mg per day.

All layers of the skin showed improvement, ranging from improvements in skin wrinkling, skin texture, age spots, moisture content, and elasticity [111]. And just like in the green algae, the pigment helps protect us from UV radiation and may reduce the chances of getting burned. So now you must be wondering, "where do I score this super supplement?" Let us have the honor of informing you.

The best source is still through eating whole foods. Astaxanthin can be found in your bright pink foods such as:

- wild-caught sockeye salmon

- krill

- crawfish

- salmon roe

- red trout

- red sea-bream

- crab

- lobster (best consumed with a glass of pink champagne followed by a piece of pink Madonna Inn cake).

Don't want to eat that much meat, or none at all, but still want the benefits and the highest bioavailability of this holy grail of antioxidants?

You can purchase supplements of astaxanthin. Just make sure it is from the algae and not synthetic. Also, make sure it's mixed with a phospholipid because it is fat soluble and mixes well with fat, increasing its absorption in your body by as much as twelve times. We love the **Dr. Mercola® Astaxanthin** because it's extracted from *H. pluvialis* algae and it is mixed with alpha-linolenic acid, a phospholipid from perilla seed oil. Thanks Doc! Another favorite source is farmed off the Kona Coast of Hawaii and manufactured by the **Nutrex Hawaii Company®**. It is known to be the best and most pure source and anything that comes from the big island gets a big aloha from us!

Just like the mirrors on the Queen Mary that have that ever so slight rosy pink hue to banish any sea sick chartreuse from your complexion, astaxanthin, when taken daily like you should, may also make you naturally turn a light shade of the most adorable pink, sans sun!

Pycnogenol® is a registered trademark name for the phytonutrient extracted from the bark of the French maritime pine tree, *Pinus pinaster*. This potent pine helps us with all the little nasties like drinking, smoking, stress and just being alive. It contains compounds that increase blood circulation, stimulate the immune system, and protect DNA from degradation. Pycnogenol® also exhibits antioxidant and anti-inflammatory effects, helping with myriad ailments. From asthma to varicose veins, from ADHD to menstrual disorders, from erectile dysfunction and male infertility to athletic endurance, Pycnogenol® ranks right up there with vitamin C as a jack-of-all-trades in the supplement world.

Speaking of which, in a study conducted in Italy, when supplementing with 100mg of Pycnogenol® the duration and severity of the symptoms of the common cold were reduced, and when taken with 200mg of vitamin C and 30mg of zinc, significant results were achieved, and the length was reduced from a week to five days (112).

That's all well and good, but what does that have to do with being more beautiful? Well, if you don't have a cold, you probably look more beautiful, because when you feel good you look good or vice versa or

something like that. Also, one of the amazing features of Pycnogenol®
is that it helps to protect skin from UV radiation [113]!

So now for all you lovelies that are going through "the change", sit
back and listen to this nugget. In a study conducted on, you guessed
it, postmenopausal women, Pycnogenol® not only increased collagen
production but also increased the production of hyaluronic acid! [114]
The participants' skin became more firm and more hydrated. There is
hope, ladies. There is HOPE. But wait... there's *more*. Let's see, what's
left? It protects your skin from UV, makes it more plump, and protects
it against the ravages of the grand climacteric... hmm... what about
hyperpigmentation? Could it be? Why, yes, it can! When these skin
studies were conducted, it was also noted that it seemed to be evening
out skin tone and reducing hyperpigmentation [113]. Well, ain't that keen
AF? If it does all of this and keeps your favorite willy working, what are
you waiting for? T-i- i-m-m-ber-r-!

Vitamin D Ahhh... the sunshine vitamin! Vitamin D can be consumed
in salmon, tuna, mackerel, and, of course, vitamin D fortified milk.
But the main source of vitamin D for your body is**...** drum roll please**,**
the sun. Yes, our bodies can actually make something, that something
being this vitamin, directly from the sun. Although, we are not plants
and cannot make our food from the sun, but neither could Audrey II.
It's a complicated biochemical reaction (aren't they all?), but basically
UVB goes in, vitamin D comes out. Voilà!, you have the vitamin that is
required to absorb calcium for proper bone growth. In addition, having a
healthy level of this vivacious vitamin can help ward off myriad diseases.
According to Dr. Jeffrey Lee, professor and chair of the Department of
Surgical Oncology at the University of Texas MD Anderson Cancer
Center in Houston, Texas, "Patients with low vitamin D levels might
be at higher risk of developing cancer, having cancer progress, or dying
of cancer, including melanoma." Say WTF? Our intention is to stop
cancer, so we don every possible form of photoprotection possible;
sunscreen, hats, gloves, and umbrellas.

We do a good job on blocking the rays, but what they didn't tell
us is that the United States is experiencing an epidemic, of sorts, of

vitamin D insufficiency [115] …which gives us skin cancer. Oh hell. The National Health and Nutrition Examination Survey indicates more than 90% of people with darker skin (including African-Americans, Hispanics and Asians), and 75% of the Caucasian population in the USA are deficient in vitamin D! [116] BTW, the melanin in our skin does a good job absorbing the rays required to make vitamin D so generally speaking, the darker the skin, the less ray penetration, and the lower the vitamin D.

Vitamin E This is a top contender for the "Antioxidant of the Year" award. As there are eight subsets of vitamin E, you may also see it listed as tocopherols (of which there are four) and tocotrienols (the other four). The tocotrienols, especially from the annatto tree, are particularly potent for their anti-inflammatory ability and are 40-60 times more effective at preventing free radical damage than the typical vitamin E supplement (alpha tocopherol). The annatto tree molecules offer the most promise for a healthy heart, anti-tumor and anti-cancer action, help with metabolic disease, osteopenia/osteoporosis, and protecting the skin. It truly is a skin-hair-nails all-in-one treatment reducing dryness and redness in skin, making hair shiny and repairing split and cracked nails.

Vitamin E is fat soluble and found in our favorite foods such as: avocados, sunflower seeds, nuts, and spinach.

Ladies, and we are particularly talking to the white women in da house. Caucasian females do not fare so well during the aging process. All of us will experience a redistribution of soft tissue, reabsorption of bone (yes – your body is eating away at your own cheekbones) and volumetric loss of fat will actually change the entire structure of your face [53]! This happens more so in white women. Wow, what a racist, misogynic thing to say! But, it's true.

You can take vitamin E internally and simultaneously slather it onto the skin. Avocado masques are cool, but we always end up eating them. Therefore, our go-to facial treatments are **Eminence®'s Citrus and Kale Potent C & E Serum** (fountain of youth in a bottle) and the luxurious **Rosehip Triple C & E Firming Oil**. These serums have this essential vitamin included to help nourish and protect.

DMAE By now, we hope you are catching on that having firm, glowing skin is going to require that you consume some healthy fats in your diet. So, while we are on the fat band-wagon, let's talk about DMAE. Dimethylaminoethanol is produced in seafood and in your brain! Without having to turn into a cannibal or brain-eating zombie, guess where you can get a solid supply of this scintilla? Ha! ?You guessed it, salmon and sardines! Anchovies and squid are other rich sources, so saddle up to the seafood buffet and enjoy these beauty-brain benefits.

DMAE is an antioxidant that helps to produce brain chemicals such as acetylcholine that are necessary to keep your mental tools sharp [117]. Improved focus, increased short-term memory and mental clarity are some cognitive enhancements linked to supplementing with DMAE. To naturally achieve increased astuteness, Dr. Perricone, a huge DMAE advocate, suggests eating salmon up to seven days per week. [118] So, fish *is* indeed a brainy food.

> DMAE offers an almost immediate tightening of the skin.

DMAE stimulates nerve function and the muscles under the skin to tighten and contract, keeping the face contoured and lifted. In a placebo-controlled study using a gel spiked with DMAE, thirty healthy young adults (ages 36-49) experienced increased skin firmness. The placebo had little or no effect while the DMAE-treated skin exhibited greater tautness [119]. Crow's feet soften, neck wrinkles appear less deep and yes, we slapped it on our elephant knees and inner thighs and felt like donning a bathing suit again.

Looking for a hydroquinone alternative to fade age spots? We thought so. Behold DMAE's membrane-stabilizing properties that: 1) help reduce the accumulation of brown pigment (lipofuscin) deposits inside cells, [120] and 2) flush excess pigment right out of affected cells [121] thus reducing those age revealing patches.

For a topical treatment, we're addicted to Swanson®'s (yes, as in the vitamin company) **DMAE Serum**. It is the fourth ingredient on the label, packed with plant extracts and when we last purchased it, cost a whopping $8.88! Slather it on everything and watch the magic begin.

Vitamin C The next superstar is vitamin C. It is often listed as ascorbic acid or tetrahexyldecyl ascorbate. Do we really need to go on about this miraculous medicine from mother nature? Ok, we will. Just make sure you are getting enough. It's not synthesized in humans, we have to consume it. There are all kinds of sources out there: oranges, red peppers and kale top the list. You can take a pill or even stir a little Emergen-C® into your water.

When applied topically, vitamin C addresses elasticity, radiance and even goes head-to-head with hydroquinone, an effective but possibly carcinogenic molecule, to reduce hyperpigmentation! Vitamin C concentrations from 0.5% to 20% show the best results, with the higher end concentrations being slightly more tingly and possibly irritating to the eyes. It's not called ascorbic *acid* for nuthin'. Just ramp up slowly (start with a few times per week) and apply serums and creams about ½ inch away from the eyes. The skin around the eyes is so thin the active ingredients will creep into that area anyway.

Vitamin C also stimulates collagen
production and makes the fibers
more stable and long lasting.

Nusgens and his colleagues reported in the Journal of Investigative Dermatology that vitamin C is required for collagen molecules to assume their functional shape. [122] Low in vitamin C? No collagen for you. To get these topical benefits, we are absolutely loving the Vitamin C **Juveel**® **Rejuvenation Treatment**. This clever company freeze-dries the vitamin C so that it remains fresh! You add the solution to the vitamin C snowballs immediately before application, guaranteeing active ascorbic acid.

Ready for a heavy dose of C? Check out **NUÅGE9®'s Soleil C Serum** with cutting edge liposomal vitamin C delivery. This helps the vitamin dive deep into the skin where it does its best work without causing irritation. This easy to apply emulsion walks the line between a liquidy serum and a cream, making it perfect to treat and hydrate at the same time. Don't go to sleep without this on your face… just sayin'. Linus Pauling, you didn't even know how right you were. Now, go eat an orange.

Green Tea Drink it, bath in it, slather it on. Kermit, it *is* easy being green. Tea is second to water as the most consumed beverages in the world. The six different types of tea (white, black, green, yellow, oolong, and post fermented) primarily come from one species: *Camellia sinensi*. The six categories are based on how much the plant wilts and the enzymes are oxidized during processing. Green tea has demonstrated favorable results in autoimmune disease [123], heart disease, [124] and the early stages of cancer including breast [125] and skin. [126]

OMG… if it's going to bat against cancer, including the big breast C, we want it and we want it now! And for the skin, studies using *in vitro* and *in vivo* animal and human skin showed its anti-inflammatory, antioxidant, photoprotective, and cancer-preventative effects after topical application and oral consumption. [127][128][129][130][131] Hello!!! Take a mindful afternoon break and sip on your anti-pollution solution. Cheers!

Collagen Sometimes it's fun to watch the beauty industry fall all over itself. We snickeringly (new word) remember when collagen was the latest craze at the yearly spa convention. Everything had collagen in it; there were collagen creams, collagen masques, collagen serums, collagen tonics, collagen-tinis, etc. Tanis stood in the middle of the crowded hall buzzing with estheticians all ablaze over these new shiny products as she loudly declared, much to Neddy's dismay, "but collagen cannot pass through the epidermis." As a hush fell over the crowd, sales reps threw daggers into Tanis from their fiery eyes and other esties screamed in dismay, Tanis felt a lot like the little tyke in "The Emperor's New Clothes" as he whispered to his father "but he hasn't got anything on." Killjoy. Well, most of the beauty industry has caught on and as much as we all wanted collagen to, not only absorb into our skin, but then integrate into the complex weave of fibers that gives us support and structure, firmness and youth, alas, it cannot.

Tanis' & Neddy's Sidebar: Absorbable Skin

Listen here people... most shit cannot absorb into our skin. We are astonished (well, actually, NOT) at the number of beauty bloggers blaring out over the worldwide web to Beware! Lest we end up with pounds of creams in our colons and blushes in our bloodstreams! It's one of those things a few of our clients say with such gusto, such conviction, such unwavering belief that everything passes directly through our skin that not even the boldest of estheticians dare correct them, until now. And to these chowder heads we say "You are wrong. Wrong. Wrong." Of course, everything does NOT pass through your skin, you ninnyhammer.

That's why nurse Betty uses a friggin' needle to poke a hole in it and why we have a mouth and digestive system to get our nutrients in... and out. What the hell is our skin for? It's a biological barrier designed to blockade as much as it can and it successfully keeps out so many harmful substances that we would probably all be dead if it did not.

If you are a molecule and want entry into epidermis land, you have to pass the four-fold challenge. Otherwise, you are stuck outside of the VIP velvet rope.

1) **Size Does Matter** There's a general understanding in the pharmaceutical world of dermatology known as the 500 dalton rule. Basically, if you are making a drug that is applied to the skin

that needs to pass through it into the system, it best be under 500 daltons or don't bother. [132] Any larger than 500 daltons and the molecule will not be able to pass through the stratum corneum layer and BAM! Your skin is effectively doing its job, acting like a wall. Now, just because some skincare ingredients are above 500 daltons does not necessarily mean they are worthless. Many do *not* have to pass through to be effective, and some are even meant to work by remaining on the top of the skin. A great example of a huge molecule that does a good job at hydrating the skin is hyaluronic acid. It is 5,000 to 20 million daltons and sits right up on top, binding water to the skin, making it plump and dewy. Another big badass molecule is collagen. It will sit on top of your skin moisturizing away waiting for your next shower only to be washed off down the drain. It can moisturize skin, but it can't increase firmness. Our favorite tiny molecules able to gain entry to the dermal layer are retinoic acid (aka our fave prescription anti-aging molecule), weighing in at 300 daltons, retinol at 286 and glycolic acid at a mere 76 daltons.

2) **Oil Versus Water** Do you melt in the rain? Ok, maybe the Wicked Witch of the West does and even though some members of the Real Housewives of Orange County might fit this bill, we are pretty sure they're puddle proof. Reason being is your skin is waterproof. It's got a lot of fat and oil in it and remember, oil and water don't mix. (Piss and vinegar, on the other hand, do.) So, oily substances will penetrate better than water-based ones... but they still have to pass the other three penetration tests. A cool example of this is glycolic acid (an alpha hydroxy acid) and salicylic acid (a beta hydroxy acid). They both pass the other tests, but glycolic is water soluble so does not penetrate as deeply as the oil soluble salicylic that sinks into pores where it fights acne.

3) **Charge!** Molecules have positive and negative electrical charges on them. Nonpolar molecules have charges pretty

evenly distributed. Agents that are nonpolar have a better chance of penetrating the skin (granted, they meet the other criteria). If one end of a molecule is more positive and another end is more negative, the molecule is polar. Water is polar and so is coconut oil. And neither of these natural ingredients are getting through your stratum corneum. But we still love them.

4) **You** The condition of the skin will matter when it comes to penetration. The skin under your eyes is much thinner than other areas, allowing for easier entry (and also possible dark circle exposure). If your skin is scratched, cut, abraded or otherwise compromised, some larger molecules may have just found their entry portal since you have a breach in your barrier. Age, temperature, moisture content and even the race of the person can all affect skin permeability. And while we're Side-barring, we do not breathe through our skin either. That's why we have lungs. We thought y'all took biology, were you sleeping? Now, back to our regularly scheduled program.

There are a couple of ways to get collagen passed through the skin barrier: inject it (go read Fillers, Freaks and Fabulousness) or swallow it! After ingestion, some studies indicate our bodies may make more collagen by a few different mechanisms (key word being "may"). This is good news since Americans spend $60.9 million a year on food, vitamins and supplements containing collagen.

But after it hits our stomach, what exactly is going on? There have been a few studies indicating that collagen production increases when it is ingested. Their results showed a statistically significant increase in skin elasticity with collagen ingestion compared to the placebo group. [133]

Based on those results, collagen supplementation is beginning to sound delicious, especially since we can add it to our morning coffee. What is even more enticing are products that mix collagen with other ingredients known to help support skin and joint health. And BTW, hyaluronic acid (HA) production is stimulated by collagen and collagen production is stimulated by hyaluronic acid. On that note, we love Collagen Complete™. A supplement that contains hydrolyzed collagen, hyaluronic acid, a couple of ingredients used by our bodies to make hyaluronic acid, and a few enzymes to help support skin health.

Hyaluronic Acid That's right folks, you can soothe joints, hydrate tissues, and at a minimum, lube your digestive tube with one big blob of berry flavored goo in your favorite beverage. We have yet to try it in a martini, but we'll be sure to make a YouTube video if we have noteworthy mixology success. Here's how it works. When taken orally, hyaluronic acid (HA) ramps up your own body's natural production of this protective polymer, presenting a non-invasive therapy for alleviating the symptoms of osteoarthritis. [134] It has also been shown that the molecules can actually be absorbed and are available to the human body [135] offering a repair system that even Jiffy Lube would be proud of.

Okay, so even though we don't believe there is one magic bullet for staying youthful, here is an interesting story that may encourage you to get your ticket for the vain train. The World Health Organization studied 990 villages and towns in Japan and reports that there are 10 times more people over the age of 85 living in the mountainous village of Yuzurihara than anywhere in North America. In 2000, ABC News sent super cool Connie Chung into Yuzurihara to unveil their secret and, by God, did she ever. These people are practically Alzheimer free, diabetes free, and cancer free (even though most work as farmers under the boiling sun sans sunscreen).

> Hyaluronic Acid boosts thick lustrous hair, wrinkle-free and spot-free skin, flexible joints and sharp vision.

Many were still farming, trimming trees and buzzing around town on their motor scooters well into their 80s... and 90s! The town doctor, Dr. Toyosuke Komori, was so damn bored, he decided to supplement his income by writing five books in the 70s and 80s about these super-agers. He had his finger on it when he attributed their youthfulness to their diet, that happened to support the body's own production of HA and was also *loaded* with HA.

When Bill Sardi, the author of "How to Live 100 Years Without Growing Old" visited Yuzurihara, now deemed "The Village of Long Life," he revealed their diet which consists of satoimo root vegetable (known as taro root or "sticky potato" even though it is *not* a potato), miso paste, dark purple sweet potato, daikon radish, buckwheat noodles, azuki bean paste (this is the red bean paste you will find in Asian desserts), and a newly introduced sticky vegetable which originated from Egypt called moloheiya. The only meat was fish caught from a local stream. [136]

We decided that since we have not been on the "Japanese Longevity Diet" since birth, we have some catching up to do. First, we are following this meal ticket to vitality as much as possible. Our local Japanese market happens to carry some of the aforementioned foods and, with a little guidance and imagination, we are Japanofying (new word) our diet. Second, we are making up for lost time and a not so perfect diet with supplements. There is scientific support that oral supplementation with hyaluronic acid is useful in maintaining skin elasticity [137] and sharp vision, [136] and providing joint support. [138] Furthermore, HA also stimulates collagen production, so you'll be plump *and* firm, just like your boobs were before 40 years of gravity. We love the liquid berry flavored HA made by **NOW**® that is easy to add to our morning smoothies. And for those of you tempted to eat your Eminence® Strawberry Rhubarb products, NOW® is the way to go for it. **Purity Products**® also makes four different HA products in capsule form, so you can pop on the run. Happy Lubing!

Biotin Pick up a bottle of a skin, hair and nails supplement and we'll bet it has biotin in it. Or at least it should. Otherwise, set that bottle right back down! Biotin is actually a B vitamin; 7, to be exact, and supports the things you imagine a B vitamin would: the metabolism of carbs and fat, neurological health, psychological function and the production of energy. B7 is also a real beauty bullet and gets its other name, vitamin H from the German words "haar" and "haut" which mean hair and skin.

Now here's another one of those things the beauty industry went zany with, biotin works when we ingest it, not when we topically apply it. Step away from all those tempting biotin shampoos and creams that promise lustrous results (unless it's a good product anyway, inexpensive, and you don't mind being lied to). We prefer boycotting these products because, well; we do mind being lied to. And one way to pull the reins in on these companies is to not buy what they're selling. We know you're smart, so let's talk about where you should be laying out the cash.

We love to start with whole foods; not the overpriced market that appears in high socioeconomic neighborhoods (did we write that out loud?), but unprocessed, hopefully unsprayed, hormone free food. When in doubt, buy wild or grow your own. Salmon and sardines (notice how frequently these fabulous fishies come up?), organ meats, egg yolks, avocados, raspberries and barley are great sources of biotin. Guess what? Those beneficial bacteria in your gut are also hard at work for you *making* vitamin B7.

Low biotin can cause brittle, weak hair and nails, hair loss, and dry cracked skin, especially around the corners of the mouth and groin (yowch). In fact, vitamin H's beauty benefits were realized when horses with dry cracked hooves were successfully treated with biotin; and after, we are sure they had a glossy pony tail in tow, too. The exact mechanism of how vitamin B7 helps with the growth of strong hair and nails is unknown, but it appears to be effective [139] and may even help skin fight off acne and fungal infections and lessen severe dryness and rashes. Giddyup.

DHEA We always recommend talking to your doctor about everything we are introducing to you in this chapter (book, really), particularly DHEA. As a matter of fact, if you are under 30, have prostate, breast or any other cancer, or you're pregnant or breastfeeding, just skip right on over this section. DHEA is not for everyone. It's not for Neddy. It may not be for you. But it's damn near a miracle supplement for Tanis, and that is how it made it into this book. And even though you can buy this little pill in your local drugstore, vitamin shop and, of course, on Amazon®, you really need to run this by your doc first; even after reading how this one supplement may help you get your mojo back, all of it, including your sex life. Here's why.

DHEA is dehydroepiandrosterone, and made by your adrenal glands, the gonads, and the brain and it is a steroid hormone. That's right, and not only is it *a* hormone but it is the *mother* of all hormones, the big daddy of bodily secretions, the grand poobah of chemical messaging. Your body can take this "pro-hormone" and make, or be stimulated to make, a shit ton of other hormones from it. These include, but are not limited to: androgens [140] such as testosterone, dihydroxytestosterone, and androstenedione and estrogens [141] such as estrone, estradiol, and estriol. These powerful sex hormones are needed for many bodily functions beyond pro-creation. They are important for maintaining high energy levels, a robust metabolism, bone, brain, and heart health. There are no natural food sources of DHEA, even though yams and soybeans are used to make "bio-identical" DHEA hormones.

> DHEA is tied to longevity, a lean, strong body and sexy bedroom antics.

And, like most good things in the human body, it begins to decline at around age 30. According to Dr. Dharmananda at the Institute for Traditional Medicine in Portland, Oregon, " at age 50, it's typically only about half the peak level, and by age 75 it declines to about 10% of the peak level." He also states that low levels in adults correlates with cardiovascular disease, breast and endometrial cancer, Alzheimer's disease, and the progression of HIV. Benefits also include decreased fat accumulation, increased bone density and energy, reduced inflammation, lessened aches and pains, and improved brain function and sex drive. So, WTF is it doing for my skin? You may be pondering. Well, put on your thinking caps, my pretties. If this is an elixir of youth, what *isn't it* doing for your beauty routine? Hell, just the fact that it helps us get out of bed, zip up our pants, and make it over to the coffeepot damn near makes us Ms. Universe and far better off than most Americans. And we've got data.

In a double-blind, placebo controlled study, 280 healthy men and women (60-79 years old) were given 50mg of DHEA or a placebo daily for a year. Bone turnover and libido improved significantly in women over 70. Improvements in skin were observed, particularly in women, in terms of hydration, epidermal thickness, sebum production, and pigmentation. The dosage did not yield harmful consequences, but normalized some effects of aging. [142] One pill, many positive effects. Yes, there's more.

We estheticians specialize in dryness, or the alleviation thereof, and that is not to exclude vaginal dryness. We are often asked by our menopausal clients if anything can be done, with no disrespect, to help lube the tube. We came across a recent randomized, placebo-controlled study on the effects of DHEA on vaginal atrophy (the thinning of the vaginal walls) and all of its related challenges such as painful intercourse, a dry and inflamed JJ, incontinence, increased UTIs (the list goes on). So, here's the good news.

All the signs and symptoms of hormone deficiencies caused by menopause can be rapidly improved or corrected by topical application of DHEA

No need for exposure to systemic estrogen. [143] It may also help with classic menopausal problems; hot flashes, cold flashes, massive insomnia, forgetfulness, weight gain, achiness, sags, bags, and wrinkles.

Not ready to take the DHEA plunge? There is a natural way to increase your levels of not only DHEA but the other fountain of youth, human growth hormone (HGH), and if you have been taking notes, you will probably guess that it is... exercise! So how much, if any, will DHEA increase after exercise in older adults? In one study with participants aged between 60-77 years old, DHEA levels were shown to significantly increase post-exercise. [144] And here is our fave. A study on the hormonal response in early postmenopausal women after high impact physical exercise revealed a 10% increase in DHEA-S levels post workout that stayed elevated for two hours. Free testosterone and estradiol increased 20%. Cortisol (the stress hormone that makes our bellies fat) decreased a whopping 36% during exercise and continued to go down another 14% post-workout! FU cortisol! Drum roll… HGH increased 80% during exercise. [145] The coolest part is that this particular exercise program used in the study was designed to help women battle osteoporosis, so it's a win-win all the way!

WHAT YOUR ESTHETICIAN **REALLY** WANTED TO TELL YOU

- Do yourself a favor and substitute that glass of wine for some pomegranate juice, you'll thank us in the morning.

- Remember to take your vitamins.

- Work with your naturopathic doctor to find out which supplements will help you accomplish your health goals. Don't have a naturopath? Find one.

- A client once told us he felt guilty about spending so much money on supplements. We told him he could only feel guilty if the word "supplement" was substituted for the word "crack."

smoke smoke

SMOKE

that cigarette

17

SMOKE, SMOKE, SMOKE THAT CIGARETTE

OR JUS' BE SMOKIN' HOT

Think this chapter is not for you? Keep reading. You smoke. And yes, we know you are smokin' hot, but you're also sucking in enough pollutants to create a negative impact on your skin and your health. Old enough to remember the Smog Alert days in the 70s? Tanis does. Remember how we stayed in from recess because the levels of ozone and pollution were burning our eyes out of our heads and made us feel like a thousand tiny knives were tearing up our lungs? Well, you smoke whether you want to or not because of the filth we are dumping into our atmosphere when we are making a bunch of disposable crap we really don't need in unregulated countries like China. But let us crawl down off of our soapbox and tell you that if you really *do* smoke, then welcome to "Smog Alert Day is every day."

In a memo posted on Berkeley Earth written by Muller and Muller, "Air Pollution kills more people worldwide each year than does AIDS, malaria, diabetes, or tuberculosis. For the United States and Europe, air pollution is equivalent in detrimental health effects to smoking 0.4 to 1.6 cigarettes per day. In China the numbers are far worse; on bad days, the health effects of air pollution are comparable to the harm done smoking three packs per day (60 cigarettes) by every man, woman, and child. Air pollution is arguably the greatest environmental catastrophe in the world today." [146] So, since we are all smokers, let's read on and see what we can do to help ourselves and find a pollution solution.

Here's something I bet your estie never told you, we know when you smoke, cigarettes, that is. Yup. And it's not just from those fumes you are emitting or those lovely stains on your teeth that your Crest® WhiteStrips aren't making a dent on. Nope. It's from your skin congestion and that unusual green-tinged oil (yes, we said GREEN) you are extruding. Although we could not find any articles supporting our observations, this topic is highly discussed in esthetician circles, but rarely shared with our clients. But for whatever reason, this grotesque phenomenon of green gooey goop occurs. It is not the main reason, or even close, to why we want you to stop smoking. It's not even for the mass destruction it is doing to your appearance.

It is because of the thousand ways (that you are already aware of) that it is detrimental to your health. We care about YOU and we don't want to terribly miss you. But if vanity will rule at the end of the day, we will be happy to talk to your inner Venus and supply you with a few narcissistic reasons you should get help, get the patch, get some gum, or go cold turkey today.

We're laying out the dermal detriments to smoking, and yes, this includes ALL of us. And if you actually smoke cigarettes or the like, just add the number of fags per day you smoke into your national average and voilà, you will know your true smoker's profile. Then, read on – and yeah –clinical research backs this data, and not some Valley Girl's Blog. Like, OMG, that's totally bitchin'.

Acne is a common skin disorder, usually considered an adolescent disease. [147] However, recent epidemiological studies have shown that it affects a significant percentage (12-14%) women between 25 and 50 years of age. [148] Post-pubertal acne is described as an inflammatory mild-moderate form, whose cause is still unknown and whose incidence is increasing. [149] Bruno Capitanio and his colleagues have discovered, however, in their clinical practice for acne treatment, a form of acne characterized predominantly by retentional lesions (micro and macrocomedones), with few inflammatory lesions (papules and pustules). This seems to be particularly frequent among adult female smokers. They named it "atypical post-adolescent acne" (APAA). Clinical evidence and experimental data showed a straight correlation between having a smoking habit and APAA. [150]

It is also commonly accepted that smoking provokes changes in skin microcirculation and nicotine induces vasoconstriction associated with local hyperaemia (blood pooling) [151] and high blood pressure. With less blood flow, your skin is not receiving as much oxygen and vitamins. You are essentially cutting off your skin's lifeline. Your skin's umbilical cord to beauty. The word "suffocation" comes to mind. So there goes your glow. Bye-bye.

With more than 4,000 nasty chemicals being delivered to your blood, you can imagine that there are at least a few hundred that damage collagen and elastin molecules. You know, those fibers holding up your face and your ass. The damage results in that amazing haggard look we are all so aware of. This could contribute to defining the "smoker's face," meaning increased wrinkling, described by several authors. [152] And of course, with all the aforementioned going on, it also delays wound healing and accelerates skin aging. [151]

Here is one last study we would rather you *not* know about. Ms. Pelle and her colleagues demonstrated that peroxidation (which BTW creates acne) is induced by cigarette smoke. [153] Their study also demonstrated that when antioxidants are applied topically to the skin, they can cause this reaction to stop happening! An average decrease of 40.9% in lipid peroxide was observed.

The good news – topical antioxidants applied to the skin really do help with environmental pollutants!

But we are not sharing this with you so that you cream up before lighting up. We still just really want you to stop smoking.

As one might imagine, the anti-pollution product marketing craze began in Asia. And where Asia leads with beauty trends, the West is soon to follow. If the product is promising to protect against the "urban effect," make sure you flip that tube around and search for vitamin C and/or vitamin A on the ingredient list. But most importantly, healthy skin that is moisturized and intact with a functional skin barrier is your best defense. Just add sunblock by day and a vitamin C serum by night and you've just created your own "city skin solution."

Now it's self-examination time. Let's start with being aware of where our stuff is being made. China, India and Saudi Arabia are on the top of the 2016 World Health Organization's list for nasty air, but before you go judging, let's point out a few other things. The USA is a top consumer of electricity and we hope you know that air pollution is directly created through our use of electricity, fuels, and transportation. Go turn off those lights!

We also cause air pollution *indirectly* when we buy goods and services that use energy in their production and delivery, which is every good and service I can think of. Seriously, stop yourself when you go to buy something new. Do you really need this? Is it possible to buy a gently used one from eBay or Goodwill? Where is it being manufactured? In a country with air quality regulations? If you broke something, can it be fixed?

Cubans are a fine example of how to appreciate and use things for a very long time. Since they practically have no new goods being produced or shipped into their country, they treat every object like a treasure. When we were in Cuba, we saw many coffee cups with handles glued back on and 1950s cars held together with bondo and duct tape. A man repairing his old fan on a balcony, shops machining parts to fix things, and women lovingly stitching clothes that need just a little TLC are just a few examples of excellent "object retention" we witnessed. Do you really need that iPhone XX? Really? And yes, the smog in China really is that bad. Tanis recently saw it floating in… when she was visiting Seoul, Korea, that is! Countries don't have walls and planets don't have spares. Mars is not an option.

Carbon dioxide (CO_2) is a good indicator of how much fossil fuel is burned and how much of other pollutants are emitted as a result. Using carbon dioxide as an indicator, the United States is the 8th leading contributor to CO_2 according to the World Health Organization. Since it is still up for debate which is worse for air quality, cars or cows (yup, that's right, cow farts plus slaughter plus refrigeration plus transportation = mega greenhouse gases), maybe it's time we all did a little more errand running on our bikes and a few less trips to Mickey D's. Aren't you glad you have an esthetician? No wonder we need so many antioxidants. Speaking of, if antioxidants are really a pollution solution, which ones are the best?

Vitamins E, C, and Green Tea top the chart and, for a plethora of golden advice, go read "Mama's Little Helpers".

WHAT YOUR ESTHETICIAN **REALLY** WANTED TO TELL YOU

- Go look at some pictures of long-term smokers. Just be smokin' hot.

- Reduce pollution and stop buying so much crap you don't need.

- Get on the anti-pollution bandwagon and get some antioxidants into your body and onto your skin. Vitamin E, C and Green Tea not only rhyme but make us fabulous.

- When Tanis was teaching high school science, she used to bring her students on a field trip to Cal State University, Fullerton, where they would examine a cadaver. This particular man had died of lung cancer. After examining the lungs, any students who had currently been smoking, quit, and those who weren't, won't. Don't be that cadaver.

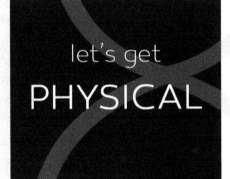

18

LET'S GET PHYSICAL

YOUR TANGO WITH EXFOLIATION

You enter a dimly lit room and there it is, waiting for you on the counter. Rough around the edges, sure, but oh baby, is it good at getting you to shed a few layers, to strip down, and possibly even blush a little... and you always look better after you've danced a steamy encounter with your... exfoliator. We're talking about your exfoliator, ladies... jeez. Because as poetic as it sounds, exfoliation is the never-ending song of life. If you're still breathing, you're shedding skin! Thus begins the "tug and pull" of a lifelong tango with your exfoliators. Even though our official discussion about flaking off is towards the end of this book, we've been touching on this topic throughout. And with all the juicy nuggets of knowledge we've blessed you with, you could practically become an esthetician yourself! But don't get any fancy ideas because we still need to pay the rent. So, this leads us to the grand finale of desquamation and we are diving deep into the world of scrubs, rubs, luffas and enzymes, something with which we all should get super friendly.

Take a moment, close your eyes, and try to remember your very first experience with... an exfoliator, that is. If you're like us, an instant flashback of a shiny-faced teenager pops up with a tube of some peachy colored kernels in hand. Yep, your dance with physical exfoliation goes *way* back. But perhaps what you didn't know was that at the same time you were reaching for that beaded concoction, you were beginning your anti-aging routine. Haven't started your two-step with exfoliation yet? Baby, you are late for the dance. Grab a partner and let's begin.

To understand exfoliation, you must first understand the anatomy of the skin and the lifespan of our precious little skin cells. Here's the thing people, we shed skin like clothes on a hot date! Humans can shed anywhere from 1 to 6 pounds of skin per year! So where is all of this sloughed off stuff coming from? Skin is made up of three layers:

1) **Epidermis**: the outermost layer of skin. It is what we see every day, provides a waterproof barrier, and creates our skin tone.

2) **Dermis**: considered our "true skin" beneath the epidermis. It contains tough connective tissue, hair follicles, and sweat glands.

3) **Hypodermis**: a deeper subcutaneous tissue made of fat and connective tissue.

Estheticians are licensed to work solely on the epidermis. Within the epidermis, there are five, let's call them "departments," through which a skin cell must pass during its lifespan. Think of it like starting an adventure in the basement of a department store and working your way to the penthouse and eventually up on the roof where you, um, fall off. Okay, maybe not the best analogy, but you get the picture. Starting from the bottom up, here are your five skin "departments:"

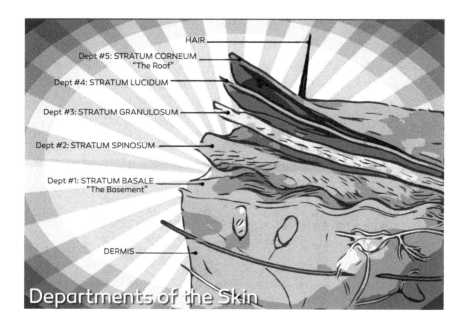

Departments of the Skin

HAIR

Dept #5: STRATUM CORNEUM "The Roof"

Dept #4: STRATUM LUCIDUM

Dept #3: STRATUM GRANULOSUM

Dept #2: STRATUM SPINOSUM

Dept #1: STRATUM BASALE "The Basement"

DERMIS

Department #1 – Stratum Basale

This is where the journey begins and little bitty cells are born; the maternity ward of your hide. Keratinocytes are formed in this "basement" layer and slowly work their way up to the higher departments of the epidermis. More on keratinocytes in a moment. Melanocytes are also found here. These are the cells that make melanin and are responsible for creating your lovely complexion and protecting our skin from the harmful effects of UV radiation. These frenemies can also make too much damn melanin, creating hyperpigmentation and melasma or mutate into melanoma.

Department #2 – Stratum Spinosum

The cells then move into this layer, which gives the skin strength and flexibility. This is where the desmosomes, the linkages between cells, are formed. They make a chain-link fence, of sorts, creating a fibrous mesh of support and structure.

Department #3 – Stratum Granulosum

This is where the party gets started when the keratinocytes begin to produce keratin (not only just a hair treatment), the main protein in the skin. The primary function of keratin is to adhere skin cells together, working as the Elmer's glue of your tissue. This keratin then attaches to desmosomes, creating a superficial protective layer.

Department #4 – Stratum Lucidum

This quirky layer is most visible on the palms of the hands, fingertips, and the soles of the feet, where the skin is thicker. It is actually a thin clear layer that gives your skin extra flexibility. Just look at the palm of your hand and stretch it wide and then relax it. See how the skin easily stretches and contracts? This is especially fun to do after eating some special brownies. Open, close, open, close, stretch, contract, stretch, contract; the pontifications are profound yet pointless. This layer also lowers the effect of friction on the skin and makes it waterproof, especially on the soles of the feet; *muy importante* if you are a Thai massage therapist or Jesus.

Department #5 – Stratum Corneum

This is the end of the line for your skin cells that started their journey in the stratum basale; it takes about 14 days for the keratinocytes to reach the penthouse of your protective armor. [154]

During their journey, keratinocytes undergo a series of biochemical and morphological changes resulting in the formation of the different layers of the epidermis. Eventually, these cells turn into the outermost layer of dead, cornified cells and form a matrix crosslinking with other proteins. This layer forms a flexible barrier that repels water and protects the body from dehydration and environmental insults. This is basically why, like OMG, everything does NOT pass directly through our skin. [155] Eventually, bonds, like the desmosomes, weaken and break and then you shed. The next time you dust, you can ponder how much of it is your own body.

The lifespan of an epithelial skin cell is approximately two to four weeks. Your cell turnover rate (CTR) is the term coined for how long it takes your skin to shed itself. Unfortunately, this rate slows down, like everything else, as you get older. What once took two weeks in infancy, takes two to three weeks as a teen, up to one month as an adult, and then suddenly plummets to every 45-90 days after the age of fifty. Happy mfkn birthday!

Approximately 25-30 layers of dead
skin cells are hanging out on our faces
at any given moment.

But there is a light at the end of this dark grey tunnel (the color of dead skin cells no matter what your ethnicity). This is where your professional esthetician comes in because there ain't nothin' better we like to do than strip. It's hard for your products to get down deep and do their best work when they are sitting on top of layers of *extra* dead skin. But exfoliation comes sashaying in to save the day! Let's show you how to do a tango kick on your skin's butt!

Our crash course on skin anatomy is complete, so let us shimmy into physical exfoliation. The directory of depilation is broken down into three categories: manual, mechanical, and enzymatic.

1) Manual Exfoliation is when you physically scrub your skin with something gritty you buy at the store, a homemade concoction, a Japanese dry brush, a luffa, or an exfoliating hand mitt… etc. This is the most common, old-school way to exfoliate. Let's call it: Entry Level Exfoliation. Many clients ask us, just how many layers of skin is a manual exfoliant sloughing off? Most people are walking around with about 20-30 extra layers of skin. The very top four layers of excess cells are called the stratum disjunction, and these are the easiest layers to remove. It's where super old ones hang out when they retire, like Florida for skin cells. Manual exfoliants help those ancient cells to "cross the rainbow" and enter cellular nirvana. It's okay to help them cross over and set them free! Manual exfoliation is great to perform one to seven times per week depending on your skin type, condition, what you are using to do the deed, and what body part you are treating.

Tanis and Neddy Sidebar: Altitude Sickness

Neddy remembers the first time she exfoliated her face. It really was a glorious experience; squeezing the tube imprinted with a picture of apricots intermingled with a scenic shot of the Swiss Alps. It seemed so cosmopolitan and she felt like she had stepped up her skincare game. The fruity aroma of what she imagined was fresh fruit combined with the grit of crushed walnuts dancing across her face with every circular motion of her pre-teen fingers. It felt like heavy duty sandpaper, but with one refreshing rinse, Voila! Her teeny bopper skin was feeling baby soft and looking brighter than ever! The beauty of a good face scrub. It was no surprise that Neddy thought this was a no-brainer and that she should scrub her face every day! Right? Wrong... so very wrong. Within days, her baby soft skin was raw, red, broken out, and peeling. She dialed back to once per week, and still her skin remained angry. So, one little girl in a pale pink coat moaned, "Lay ee odl lay ee odl lay OOH OOH."

What poor little Neyney didn't know was that she was committing exfoliation hari kari. In fact, OG cult classic St. Ives° Apricot Scrub, has gotten into some very hot water, and is now facing a lawsuit of Judge Judy proportions! This is a 2016 class action lawsuit and the plaintiffs claim two things: 1) that the crushed walnut powder creates microscopic tears in the skin, exposing it to infections and irritation, and 2) that it's *not* noncomedogenic as the label implies (meaning it *does* clog pores). The jury is still out on this case, with people drawing a line in the sand and picking sides.

Our research reveals that St. Ives° contains sodium lauryl sulfate (SLS), an ingredient detailed in the chapter "Buy Cheap, Break Out." This strong surfactant often strips the skin of its natural sebum, drastically affecting the skin barrier function, turning your once moisture rich skin into a barren desert. All of this scratching and irritation can weaken the stratum corneum, giving way to even more potential problems. Another doozy, St. Ives° contains preservative methylchloroisothiazolinone (MCI) which is almost always found with its partner in crime, methylisothiazolinone (MI). MI was rated in 2013 by the American Contact Dermatitis Society as "Allergen of the Year." [156]

Yeah kids, this is some real deal Holyfield combination here! In fact, around 2% of the population has shown an allergic reaction to this preservative. If you have sensitive skin conditions like acne, rosacea, or eczema... RUN to the other side of the dancefloor! Yes, we all have different skin types and conditions that react differently, so there will always be super models like Gigi Hadid still swearing by this classic. With Glamour magazine naming it one of the "Best Exfoliators Under $10" back in 2013, it's no wonder many still use this guilty pleasure. But, with so many advancements in the world of manual exfoliants, it is time we retire this with our cassettes and Aqua Net°. Here's the skinny. It's not that the Swiss Alp ingredients don't work, it's that they work a little too aggressively for the precious skin on your mug. Do we hate you St. Ives°? No. No, we don't. We will happily scrub our feet, backs and buttocks with you until the end of time. But don't come near our faces!

Speaking of the advancements in the world of scrubs, breakthrough ingredients are dipping into the scene and revamping our spa experiences. Fun and exotic components like volcanic clay, Aztec amaranth, grated coconut, and coffee beans are some of the new chicos on the block. Flashy though they may seem, these newbies, along with others, are bringing some awesome added benefits to our daily regimens. From improving fat absorption, to removing toxins, and adding hydration and antioxidant boosts, this new class of manual exfoliants are more than one trick ponies!

What we adore about manual exfoliants is that you can use them and even make them yourself! It really is the "self-empowerment" tool in the world of skincare. Do it yourself recipes are plentiful online; our fave base ingredients are pink Himalayan salt and coconut sugar.

Look for manual exfoliants featuring very fine particles. The smaller the granule, the more effective the exfoliation.

Teensy bamboo particles work to polish skin and smooth spheres made from the seed of the desert jojoba shrub are usually a good bet. For the face, we have been enthusiastically recommending **Pharmaskincare® Botanica Vit Complex Exfoliant** since 2005. It cleanses, it exfoliates, it combats breakouts like nobody's business, and we personally use it every damn day.

For the body, we are obsessed with the luffa (not loofah). A luffa is a natural sponge that does not come from the ocean but from a gourd! Tanis' dad introduced us to the **Luffa Farm** in Nipomo, California. It's one of the only places in the USA that not only grows this glorious gourd, but does so using heirloom seeds. Their luffas are ridiculously soft and are even face-friendly. The farm gives free tours and has the most adorable gift "hut" where you can find luffas of all shapes and sizes, handmade soaps, soaps with luffas inside, essential oils, bath soaks and all kinds of skincare delicacies. The staff are super friendly, knowledgeable and passionate about all things luffa. If you can't make it out to the farm, you can visit their website at www.theluffafarm.com. So scruba-dub and brusha-brush amigos!

2) **Mechanical Exfoliation** is when you physically exfoliate your skin with the aid of a machine. The best and most effective example is microdermabrasion. This is a minimally invasive procedure used to renew overall skin tone and texture. It can improve the appearance of sun damage, wrinkles, fine lines, age spots, acne scarring, melasma, and other skin-related concerns and conditions. There are two different

microdermabrasion machines: 1) powdered aluminum oxide crystals are shot at the skin (think sandblasting) or 2) a diamond encrusted head is dragged across the epidermis (think sandpapering). Both use a vacuum to hold the heads tight against the skin as they are pulled along the surface. The vacuum simultaneously sucks up dead skin cells and grime. People who have high capillary activity, with lots of vessels near the surface of the skin, may not be candidates because the suction may cause the capillaries to rupture.

A study to analyze the effects of aluminum oxide crystal microdermabrasion was performed on 10 individuals with photo damaged skin. The subjects received one treatment per week for five or six weeks. A physician analyzed the skin along with a self-assessment by the participants. The docs noted some decrease in skin stiffness and an increase in smoothness and vascular activity (possibly from the suction). Seven out of 10 patients noted a mild improvement. [157]

We both utilize diamond head microdermabrasion in our practices (avoiding the use of crystals, which can be inhaled, particularly by the person receiving the treatment). We are careful not to make promises of reduced acne scarring (if the scar is deep into the dermal layer) or a drastic reduction in hyperpigmentation or acne. We know from experience that it usually takes more than just micro to get these goals accomplished, but we love it to jumpstart a person's exfoliation game and create some instantly gratifying glow.

3) Enzymatic Exfoliation is the use of proteins from pineapples and papayas to aid in decortication. Enzymes are proteins that speed up reactions. Bromelain (in pineapples) and papain (in papayas) are what may help the plants form seeds. On our skin, these enzymes act like Pac-Mans that rove around chomping up the proteins of dead skin. They help to break the bonds between amino acids, the building blocks of proteins, essentially making them fall apart. That's why you can often feel a tingle in your mouth and on your lips when you are eating these tropical wonders; these flesh-eating fruits are getting a little cannibalistic and eating you right back! But not to worry, these enzymes aid in food digestion and reduce bloating and inflammation in the body. They can be used in cooking to tenderize meat and bromelain is often ingested to help with arthritis pain, sprains, and bruises. It is also being analyzed as a potential anti-cancer agent because in one study, women that ingested bromelain started to produce cells that targeted and killed breast cancer cells. [158]

When we estheticians heard about some enzymes that are "flesh-eating" and can be used to tenderize meat, we immediately pondered the outcome of putting them on our face. Would they tenderize our faces, too? By golly, it does. These enzymes are excellent at exfoliation by breaking down keratin fibers in the skin. When the removal of dead cells is accelerated, so is the repair and renewal of the skin. Collagen production and the stimulation of fresh healthy cells also increases. Since the enzymes provide anti-inflammatory benefits while helping to unclog pores, they are good for problematic and even sensitive skin. **Shira®** **Shir-Organic Pure Pineapple Papaya Enzyme Peel** feels and smells like a cool jelly-like piña colada mask. But behold the results! We love it because it hydrates while simultaneously dissolving dead skin, leaving it supple and radiant. For a powerful punch from a combo of exfoliants, try **ExPürtise® Effective Anti-Aging Enzyme Peel**. It combines a fruit enzyme complex with glycolic and lactic acids (chemical exfoliants addressed in "Peel It Off and Start Over") with a cacophony of plant extracts to soothe and protect against free radicals. This zero down-time treatment will not cause intense redness or post peeling, but it does reduce signs of aging while promoting a more youthful appearance. This product won the "2018 Aesthetician's Choice Award" for a damn good reason!

WHAT YOUR ESTHETICIAN
REALLY WANTED TO TELL YOU

- Tired of your dull, drab skin? So are we. Please exfoliate.

- Most people have about 20-30 extra layers of dead, gray skin, so pick up a scrub, luffa, or even your old pair of cords from the 70s but for f*ck's sake, manually exfoliate.

- Mechanical exfoliation involves a machine, like a microdermabrasion machine, that can jumpstart your way to a smoother, even complexion.

- Carmen Miranda was onto something. Attack your fruit basket and discover the benefits of enzymatic exfoliation. Gentle enough for even the most sensitive skin, so samba, tango, and waltz your way to smoothness. Olé!

peel it
OFF
and start over

19

PEEL IT OFF AND START OVER

AHA'S, BHA'S, AND OTHER THINGS THAT BURN

About 15 years ago, Tanis had another brilliant idea. She gave herself a chemical peel right before heading up to northern California for a little R&R. Now, we're not talking about some pansy-ass organic fruit acid peel, but a full-blown modified Jessner's Peel that she had painstakingly and painfully applied three days prior to the trip. That meant, about the time she was rolling into Carmel by the Sea, her face had turned from a Sex in the City Samantha red to a nice shade of baby shit brown including chunks of flesh that were flapping in the wind.

Upon entering a rest stop bathroom to, er, get some rest, a line of ladies stared at her face and then excitedly inquired if she had on a mud mask and noted that it was cracked and peeling. Tanis quickly explained to them that it was actually her *face* falling off, she was hoping to find a cuter one underneath. No luck. But what emerged was more smooth, pink and rosy, radiant skin!

Healthy skin renews itself about every 28 days... for teens. If you're middle aged, it's between 28-42 days and for those of us over 50, we could be waiting up to 84 days for new cells to appear on the scene. The older cells on the surface build up and eventually are pushed off as the new cells underneath mature and rise to the top. Our outermost organ is trying to shed about 30,000-40,000 dead cells per minute. That's up to 8.8 pounds of dermis per year! Just don't get too excited, new cells immediately replace the old ones and your weight is maintained. UV exposure also slows down the renewal process and leads to a nasty accumulation of dead skin cells that are gray in color. Thus, the term "ashy," that is often used for complexions that need to get their exfoliation game on.

So, what is a chemical peel? Neddy remembers watching a horror movie when she was a kid that involved a scene in a hospital where the evil doer picks up a bottle of phenol and throws it at the unsuspecting victim. As Neddy watched the horrified man's face melt into a puddle on the floor, little did she know she was watching the workings of one of the first facial peeling agents! Heavy. Phenol, along with resorcinol, trichloroacetic acid (TCA), and salicylic acid were being used by dermatologists as early as the 1800s. Needless to say, chemical peels have come a long way, baby, and phenol has even been banned in Canada and Europe and is used primarily to make plastics, strip paint off your walls, and the like. Needless to say, Neddy steers clear of "the puddle maker."

Chemical exfoliation is a process that involves controlled injury to the skin's natural protective barrier.

The skin is forced to repair itself and new cells with more collagen and elastin are produced. They eventually rise to the surface to make their shining debut, oh behold the glory! Since most people are walking around with about 30 extra layers of dead skin, their removal helps increase penetration of all those fabulous products you are spending a shit ton of money on. Instead of sitting on top of layers of crusty cells, the products can actually get down to the deeper layers where they do their real work.

You'll want your professional esthetician or doctor to treat your skin with higher concentrations of acids that would most likely cause your skin to visibly flake or peel. Not only will they be trained on how to monitor the acid's activity level, but they will also know how to prepare the skin and quickly neutralize the acid. Your esthetician or doctor will most likely want to see you before the treatment day to decide which peel will be best to attain your skin goals. You will need to adhere to a list of dos and don'ts starting about two to three weeks before the actual peel. You should receive specific pre-and-post-peel directions including how to cleanse and care for the skin after the treatment.

Unfortunately, some people are so irresponsible and greedy that they are posting professional strength peels for sale on the internet. You may think you've hit the chemical peel jackpot if you find some of these offerings, but don't be tempted to save a few bucks, buy the peel on line, and risk burning, discoloring, and generally messing up your face. You are way too smart for that nonsense.

Lucky for us, the days of harsh chemical peels are somewhat "retro" as data steers technology towards less inflammatory and more effective ways to peel off the old. What this means in the spa industry is that less strong chemical peels are being applied in the treatment room as estheticians teach their clients how to decorticate the dermis in the privacy of their own powder rooms. There are even low dose at home "leave on" peels that have hit the scene, such as **Arbonne Intelligence® Genius Pads** and **Eminence® Exfoliating Peels** that are targeted towards specific skin conditions. These are swiped on the skin before bed and specifically treat hyperpigmentation, breakouts, aging skin and, yes… even sensitive skin! Swipe, sleep, treat. There really is an acid for everyone.

In addition to the physical scrubs and enzymatic action described in the chapter "Let's Get Physical", we will now delve into the wonderful world of acids because there is definitely more than one way to skin this cat. Meow.

Face-Worthy Acids:

Alpha Hydroxy Acids

Alpha hydroxy acids (AHAs) are a group of organic carboxylic chemicals that can be naturally occurring or made in the lab. The most common AHAs used in the cosmetic industry and their natural sources are glycolic (from sugarcane, pineapple, beets and grapes), lactic (from sour milk and tomato juice), malic (from apples), mandelic (from bitter almonds), tartaric (from grape wine) and citric (from citrus). BTW, even though both citric acid and ascorbic acid (vitamin C) come from citrus fruit, they are different molecules. Citric acid may be used to adjust the pH of skin care products and ascorbic acid is typically used for its anti-aging benefits.

Alpha hydroxy acids were "rediscovered" in the late 1980s for their anti-aging benefits, but they were unknowingly used by early civilizations to enhance the appearance and health of skin. Cleopatra was the sole female of the ancient world to rule alone and control the largest territory; she could alleviate a famine, build a fleet, suppress an insurrection… all while rocking her beauty routine, which probably included AHAs! Sour milk (lactic acid) was used by noble Egyptians as part of their skin rejuvenation regimen. Ancient Romans made masques from the sludge on the bottom on wine barrels (tartaric acid). In the middle ages a feast goer that was served old, nasty wine and ended up wearing more than they drank may have been heard proclaiming upon awakening from their liquor lobotomy, "That fusty wine that spillith upon me wast not fit for consumption, but it gaveth me glowing skin!"

French courtesans caught on and saved bottles of party leftovers for cosmetic uses. Hell, the ancient Indians and Turks used to use piss and fire to illicit the same cellular response that AHAs have on the skin! But tiki torches and golden showers aside, how do these awesome acids act on the epidermis? It is theorized that alpha hydroxy acids remove calcium ions from the cell adhesions by chelation, causing a disruption in the cadherins of the desmosomes and adherens junctions, resulting in desquamation. [159] WTF? Simply stated, AHAs penetrate deep into the dermal layer of skin loosening the "glue" that holds dead skin cells together so that they can easily fall off. Exfoliation not only helps to stimulate faster production of new skin, but it helps to unclog pores, which makes AHAs excellent ingredients to help combat breakouts.

Often overlooked are the other amazing benefits of AHAs, such as the increased stimulation of fresh collagen and elastin production. Collagen and elastin are the architecture of our skin, making it firm, toned, and give it that "bounce back" quality of baby skin. AHAs also acts as a humectant, drawing water deep into the dermal layers, making it plump and moist.

Glycolic Acid Each AHA has its own slightly unique attributes, but glycolic acid is the Queen of AHAs offering the most anti-aging benefits. This is primarily due to its small molecular weight. We always knew size does matter, and in this case, the smaller the better. These minute molecules can penetrate deeply where they do their best work. Stronger glycolic acid peels ranging from 20% to 70%, are typically performed once or twice per year; an older trend since they can trigger skin inflammation, increasing the chance of hyperpigmentation and scarring. These are being replaced with lower-level peels (5%-10%) that you can have performed during facials. Or, you can perform them at home more consistently, which seems to yield even better results without the injury.

New studies indicate that the benefits of glycolic acid go beyond the obvious. Treatment of the skin with 2% glycolic acid helps to protect it from the damaging effects of UVB. There is less inflammation and DNA damage in the treated skin compared to untreated skin. [160] The kooky thing is that it can simultaneously increase your sensitivity to solar exposure, [161] so the trick is to use products that contain glycolic acid and then block yourself from the sun (we know that you already do that).

In addition to the percentage of acid, the pH of the product plays a role in the availability and, therefore, the performance of a product containing glycolic acid. Too much acid availability and you are going to get red and peely, too little and you're in the land of da nada – no exfoliation, no glow, no nothing. An ideal pH range is between 3-4 but this is rarely listed on the package, so what's a skin junkie to do?

Sometimes, the "patch test" or trusting someone, like your professional esthetician, is the best way to tell. Patch test the product on your skin and you should feel a gentle tingle for a few seconds. Do expect a little instant gratification. An effective product makes you look refreshed after application, possibly with a little glow. Our favorite AHA night treatment is the **Peony Perfecting Dream Cream by NUÅGE9**®. It delivers an effective 10% punch of glycolic acid and is laced with other brightening agents such as Peony, Pineapple, and Passionflower, and the price is about half *less* than many AHA creams! Beauty on a budget... brainy!

Lactic Acid This is another AHA making a splash on the acid scene. According to Global Market Insights, lactic acid use will demonstrate the largest growth in the beauty industry between 2016 and 2024. Lactic acid is naturally occurring in our bodies in our sweat, and is generated during intense exercise (that's the "burn" you feel during squats and while running full speed to be first in line to ride Pirates of the Caribbean). We love it because it is very user friendly and safe for almost everybody. The molecule is larger than glycolic acid so it does not penetrate as deeply, delivering a gentler exfoliation. Lactic is also a good humectant hydrating the skin while simultaneously providing antimicrobial benefits and suppressing melanin production. We are totally loving **Eminence**®**'s Mangosteen Daily Resurfacing Concentrate**; light, tropically aromatic, with a hint of lactic. They also make a professional peel containing mangosteen infused with 10% acid that you can have applied by your esthetician.

Mandelic Acid derived from bitter almonds, is finding its way into more products. Again, like lactic, it's bigger than glycolic, twice as big, and is slower to penetrate, making it less irritating than its AHA cousin. It helps with breakouts and the hyperpigmentation that often accompanies pimples on darker skin.

Mandelic Acid is a solid choice
for melanin rich skin such as
African and Indian.

Melanin rich skin is often sensitive skin and beta hydroxy acids (such as salicylic) that are typically preferred for blemish blasting, can sometimes be too drying for this skin type. Glycolic can be too irritating. But gentle mandelic acid presents as a possible pimple slayer that also helps hinder hyperpigmentation. Dark skin is more prone to ingrown hairs and folliculitis (the inflammation of hair follicles usually by bacteria or fungus), and mandelic acid is a real workhorse combating microorganisms while helping to prevent ingrowns. The synergistic blend of lactic and mandelic can prove to be a potent cocktail treating acne, discoloration, razor burn, ingrown hairs and large pores! We adore USA made **AlmondClear**® products that include washes and serums formulated specifically for the body or face. We have used them to help clear biker's butt (a rash that can develop on cyclists' heinies) and keratosis pilaris (on the upper arms). Thanks AlmondClear®, for delivering bump free buttocks to a triathlon near you.

If AHAs are all the holler... why isn't EVERYONE using them? Well, we were wondering the same thing. Perhaps the benefits are just unknown to consumers or they are confused about which type to use, their strengths, or applications. They may also increase sensitivity in the skin, especially during the first three months of use. A slow ramp up is recommended and, of course, always wear sun protection. Also, when using any new product, a patch test (usually on the inner wrist) is recommended to determine if you have an allergy (as opposed to just a sensitivity). And of course, if you are already on a topical such as a vitamin A derivative (Retin-A® or retinol), discontinue use or consult your doctor before beginning AHAs. Then you will be ready to experience an ancient acid in modern applications delivering lasting results!

Beta Hydroxy Acids

Beta hydroxy acids (BHAs) are another group of organic carboxylic chemicals. The superstar of this syndicate is the sensational salicylic acid. Humans have been on to the miracles of this molecule since the Assyrians and Sumerians were stocking it in their plant "pharmacies" back in 4,000 and 3,500BC! Even way back then, they had figured out that the bark of the willow tree was working some medicinal magic because guess what… it contains salicin, the natural plant form of aspirin! Oh yes, my friends, imagine being an ancient Assyrian with an aching cavity or some righteous menstrual cramps and *not* being able to walk over to your medicine cabinet and pull out some Advil® or oxycodone. We know you would be standing beside us gnawing on that friggin' bark like a beaver at the Dam Design Academy. Hell, we probably would have built our house, furniture and eating utensils out of that wood so we could just chew on a bedpost or candlestick to receive some migraine, childbirth, or hangover relief. Nom-nom.

Salicylic Acid Willow bark powder was the snow blow of BC and is still in use today as a natural alternative to lab-created aspirin. As you may have already figured out, salicin converts to our beloved salicylic acid. That beautiful bark not only relieves pain, but it's also found in beauty products. The industrial scale production of salicylic acid began in 1874 by German chemists and has been in use as a peeling agent for about 2,000 years, recently mainstreaming right into a gazillion over-the-counter acne products. Like AHAs, salicylic acid can be used in higher concentrations to create injury to the skin, causing it to peel and replenish. It has anti-inflammatory properties and self-neutralizes on the skin, making it a user-friendly excoriating agent. Since it has such good keratinolytic properties (breaking the fibrous keratin in the epidermis), it is used to help get rid of dandruff, scaly psoriasis, and in higher doses even warts! Even though we have set you straight about how not everything can pass through your skin barrier, salicylic acid actually can. We are going to relay two horror stories to you just so you will never find yourself wildly and mindlessly misusing salicylic acid.

We don't want to scare you off since it helps so many people, especially with breakouts, but we just want you to buy low dose cosmetic products and use them according to the instructions on the package... like you always do.

Horror story #1: A dude with psoriasis applies a 40% (WTF?) salicylic ointment to about 41% (again, WTF?) of his body. Already you should be going... holy shit! That's a lot of really strong acid to be pouring over almost half your friggin' body. Red flags, people. Yes, it's way too strong over way too much of his body and yes, it absorbs and yes; he spends 14 days in the hospital undergoing hemodialysis. [162]

Horror story #2: A 36-year-old woman was hospitalized with fever, sudden deafness and severe metabolic acidosis after treating her psoriasis with a 10% salicylic acid ointment for four days. [163] She recovers, but there have been deaths. We share these horror stories because we actually saw that you can purchase these higher strengths (even 60%) on the internet! We guess they're probably to burn off one little wart, but they're out there, so be aware. If you are interested in treating your face to a salicylic acid peel, please contact an experienced doctor or esthetician to perform your peel.

Time to focus on the unbelievable benefits of this BHA when appropriately used for <u>cosmetic</u> purposes according to the package instructions. You've already learned it can penetrate into the skin and in very low concentrations. This is great because it helps remove dead cells lodged deep inside of follicles; something that AHAs don't do very well. In gentle formulations with willow bark extract, the products can even calm and soothe angry skin. Salicylic can also reduce pore size and we have had amazing results on older, menopausal skin that is breaking out and rapidly losing its elasticity. One client had such tight, clear, radiant skin we thought she had some other radical treatment performed, but she was simply using our recommended **Arbonne® Clear Future Corrective Acne Pads** (clearly, not just for acne)! Using salicylic acid as a breakout preventer is great, but we still recommend 5% benzoyl peroxide for spot treating pimples. It works more quickly than salicylic to combat a blemish, but keep it right on the pimple because it can be irritating and drying.

Other Note-Worthy Acids

Trichloroacetic Acid (TCA) Among the most widely used peeling products in skincare, TCA is used in a range of concentrations to deliver different peel depths. A professional TCA peel can stimulate collagen production and improve textural inconsistencies, leaving skin more firm and smooth.

Retinoic Acid aka vitamin A or tretinoin, retinoic acid is an excellent way to continually "peel" and rejuvenate skin. It is a critical component of eliminating hyperpigmentation (you will find more about vitamin A in the chapter "Look On the Bright Side"). But whether or not you have hyperpigmentation, vitamin A will be your best bet for cell renewal and can be used as a standalone peeling agent or (carefully) with other exfoliating chemicals. Your esthetician will help guide you in incorporating this miracle worker into your skin regimen.

We call retinoic acid a vitamin, but it is actually a topical hormone that controls growth and other important functions in our cells. When you go in the sun, your vitamin A levels decrease about 10-15% in about 45 minutes. You may think you can eat your levels up higher by increasing the amount of vitamin A in your diet, but unfortunately, it doesn't work quite like that. If you wanted to consume food to get your levels back to normal, you would have to stay in a cave and eat carrots and cantaloupes for a week! Otherwise, topical supplementation will be your most efficient method to feed your skin this critical nutrient.

If you use retinoic acid as your primary peeling agent, you are employing the best skin solution "two-fer" in the industry. Not only does vitamin A help the skin exfoliate rapidly (yes, you will have to contend with some flaking and peeling when using this acid), but it also helps to rebuild the tissue! It combats all the evils of photo-aging, helping to keep the layers of tissue compact and the skin moist. It reduces levels of pigmented lesions. Retinoic acid maintains collagen and elastin levels and keratinocytes remain healthy with intact DNA and a reduction in the chance of cancer! It acts as your skin's demolition crew *and* construction crew delivering a new youthful facial facade!

Breaking News Beyond the tried-and-tru- classics, there is an assembly of new acids, unique blends, and designer formulations that ward off wrinkles and deliver pro-youth results! Flower acids from hibiscus and lotus root, co-mingling vitamin A with peptides, and fun and effective "wine" products containing tartaric acid are some of the new couture formulations that you may want to check out. Let us know if you find any faves... we are sure you will!

WHAT YOUR ESTHETICIAN **REALLY** WANTED TO TELL YOU

- If it's been in the beauty industry for 6,000 years, it works. Take a lesson from our girl, Cleo. Go retro and try some acid.

- Know your numbers. Acids can be your new BFF or your worst enemy. Purchase retail products from a professional and use according to package directions.

- Less is more. Weaker acids applied more frequently deliver results with less inflammation. Explore at home peels for anti-aging, acne clearing and brightening benefits.

- Try something new! Mandelic for melanin-rich beauties and fun designer formulations offer unique options and effective results.

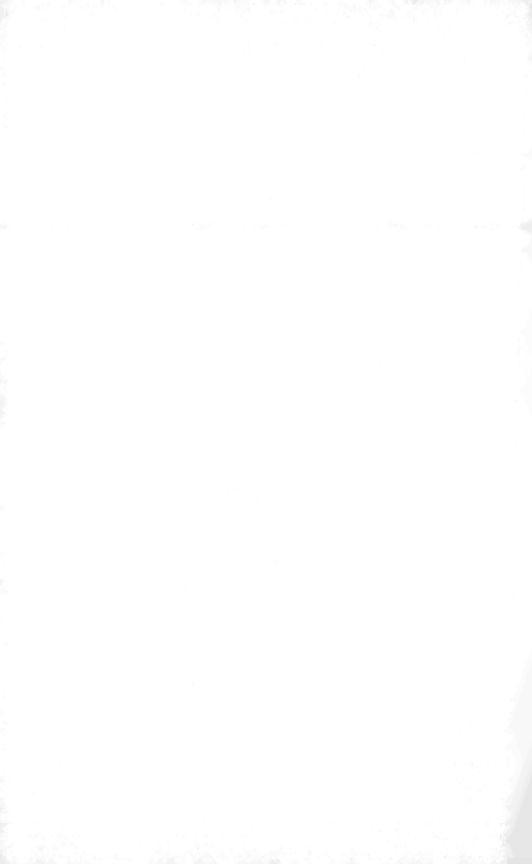

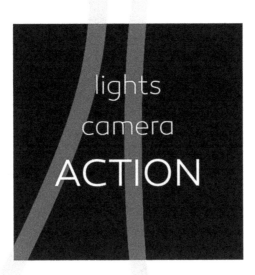

20

LIGHTS, CAMERA, ACTION

LEDS, IPLS, AND ULTRASONIC

A traditional facial is a wonderful thing, always has been, always will be. There is nothing that can replace an hour of soothing, yet seriously focused attention on the one thing that everybody's looking at, your face. It is a sacred ceremony that covers all the skincare basics; steaming, cleansing, exfoliation, and extractions ending in a grand finale of whipped delicacies and potent serums being mindfully massaged into your magnificent mug. If you had to choose between a facial or another technological based service, such as the ones we are about to explain, we would recommend the facial. It is the mainstay for healthy, clear skin and without that, we don't give a damn how many LEDs, IPLs, lasers, tasers or whatever the latest rave is you've got aimed at your head. Heed our advice, and build your beauty routine upon the foundation of the professional facial, and all other treatments will be cherries on top! Speaking of which, let's ride the wavelengths of light and electricity to a firmer, more fabulous future. Beam us up, Scotty!

LEDs Yup, we were at another skin convention when Tanis managed to embarrass the shit out of Neddy, again. LED had just hit the scene and every vendor under the sun was selling devices and touting their results. It firms your face! It makes your collagen grow! It clears acne! It relieves pain! "It sounds like this year's snake oil," Tanis grumbled as they meandered down aisle after aisle of sales people, albeit *gorgeous* sales people, waving light sabers around everyone's heads.

"This is what it would look like if Darth Vader and Han Solo had become estheticians," Tanis would snicker to herself; the ever Doubting Tanis.

"Then go ask them for the data," Neddy finally yelled, sick of the Debbie Downer 'tude and the useless bitching. So Tanis did. And the response was even more annoying than the bitching. NASA developed it! It was used to grow plants in space! It is FDA approved! First, Tanis was happy to remind them that the FDA does not "approve" devices as if to say they put their five star stamp of approval on it and that it will most certainly deliver every beauty claim that the sales people were happy to convey to us. The FDA does "clear" devices, though, so we were happy that the devices won't actually burn out our eyes or are programmed by the Chief to Self-Destruct at the termination of Agent 99's first treatment. Tanis informed them that at no time in the foreseeable future was she and Neddy planning on becoming astronauts with a botany bend and were going to begin their own "Plants, In, Space" series. So, "Show me the data!" soon became Tanis' mantra as soon as someone unwittingly mentioned LEDs. Until... the day she saw the data... then everything changed. Light-emitting diodes (LEDs) were actually first developed in 1927 by a Russian inventor with no formal education or research positions, but yet, he followed his passion to become the Superfly scientist of semiconductors! [164] Oleg Losev figured out how the hell these light-emitting diodes worked, and then pegged some practical uses for them.

So how do they work? Simply stated, an LED converts electrical energy into light energy, and the color comes from the diode itself, not some painted-on coating or bulb. And yes, in the late 1980s, NASA studied how LEDs could grow plants in space. I guess the astronauts had other ideas for the hand-held wands of mesmerizing glow because somehow, when the space shuttle landed, NASA also announced that the LEDs that had been shot off into deep space for plant growth also helped to ease pain and stimulate cell rejuvenation in the astronauts. We're not sure which one of you was the first to hold the WARP-10 LED device against your aching back, but we are sure glad you did! And we won't mention how fabulously firm your faces looked at the end of your mission. NASA job perks.

Tanis' and Neddy's Sidebar: Leave A Light On

Did you realize that most of the light emitted by the sun is invisible? Light travels in waves and the length of these waves is measured in nanometers (friggin' small units of measurement). The longer the wavelength (700nm-1 millimeter), the lower the frequency and energy. These are infrared waves, microwaves, and radio waves and they are invisible. The shorter the wavelength (0.01-400nm), the higher the frequency and energy. Examples are UV rays, X-rays, and gamma rays (from our martian space guns, of course) and they are invisible as well. These are the most harmful, and can alter DNA and damage the deeper layers of skin. The wavelengths that we *can* see are the medium waves (400-700nm); when we look at a rainbow, we see all the wavelengths in this visible range of light. The skin industry is interested in both the visible forms of light, as we experience it from LEDs, and also the invisible since excess UV rays can damage our tissue while infrared waves, which we experience as warmth from the sun, help reduce muscular pain and aid in the penetration of some products. Just a few reasons to get illuminated about light!

When skin is exposed to LEDs of different wavelengths, different positive outcomes are realized in the skin. The first trick is to plug in your hand-held device at a place where you find yourself resting every day.

Perhaps it is near the couch, so when you are binge watching The Big Bang Theory, you can treat your skin at the same time. No time for the telly? Leave it on your nightstand, so when you curl up with your favorite book at the end of the day, like the one you are holding, you can simultaneously reverse the signs of aging. So like exercise, if you're not getting your LED groove on a daily basis, you may not actually see results. With that being said, we encourage our clients to buy a device to bring home and use daily instead of throwing their money away with single, high price tag treatments, performed at a money grubbing spa. Just sayin'. This technology has been supported by so many studies that the question is not really *if* it will work for you, but *how long* will it take to work for you. Manufacturers suggest using the device 3 minutes per area, 5-7 days per week. In about two months, or sometimes much sooner, when it comes to treating acne, you are going to notice marked improvement in your skin. And then, just like exercise, you keep going. Now you understand why a one-shot deal in a spa is not cutting the mustard. Shame on those people for taking your hard- earned money. They probably used it to buy their own personal home LED device. BTW, the cost to buy your own quality LED saber is about $150-$250; about the cost of ONE treatment in some spas. Let's break down LEDs according to wavelength to find out which lights are going to help you check off your skin care goals. This is where that data Tanis was so feverishly searching for comes into play.

Red LED These wavelengths of light are the anti-aging LEDs and you would be smart to incorporate them into your daily skincare regime. So, you may think, yeah, yeah, I already know how acids and retinoic acid can help stimulate collagen and new cell growth and cellular repair; I've already got this covered. But there is a big BUT here people. This modality does not depend on traumatizing the skin to elicit a healing response! Au contraire mon frère! This method is "atraumatic" meaning the skin does <u>not</u> have to be damaged before the miraculous makeover begins! No redness. No downtime. No weird side effects. That means you can begin using LED light at any time, even when we are approaching red carpet season or holidays with the in-laws. Studies show that red light activates fibroblast growth factor, increases type I pro-collagen, and decreases the enzyme MMP-1 that breaks down collagen[165][166][167]

Let us repeat… it stimulates new cells with increased collagen while simultaneously slowing down the enzyme that destroys our precious collagen! Do you hear us? Making collagen… increased. Breaking collagen… decreased. Now you are beginning to understand why you need to bring one of these bad boys home and have a nightly rendezvous with your magic wand. Use of red LED reduces bruising and swelling after plastic surgery, [168] helps to speed up wound healing after laser treatments, [169] and people experience significantly improved skin complexions and skin texture. 80.4% of users give it a thumb's up! [170] Behold the benefits of red LED:

• Anti-aging and regenerative effects.

• Increases rate of healing.

• Increases collagen production.

• Decreases the enzyme that breaks down collagen.

• Increases circulation.

• Improves even skin tone and texture.

Blue LED Got acne? Get a blue LED light, pronto. Tremblay and his research buddies gave patients with mild-to-moderate inflammatory acne two 20-minute treatments of blue LED per week for 4 to 8 weeks. Ninety percent of patients were satisfied with the result. [171] These patients had a 50% reduction in lesion counts and nine patients completely cleared! Two similar clinical studies showed reductions in lesion size, number, and erythema in patients as evaluated by themselves and a doctor after treatment with blue LED. [172][173] Neddy shipped a blue LED device to her nephew with instructions that he should use the light as much as possible; while reading, studying, watching American Horror Story, etc. Against every esthetician bone in her body, she did *not* encourage him to change up his skin care routine, or lack thereof, or his habit of eating pizza three times daily. Even though he was experiencing level III acne at the onset of Neddy's at-home experiment, her nephew quickly cleared and was downgraded to a category I by doing nothing more than waving the blue wand. Behold the benefits of blue LED:

- Kills *P. acnes*, the bacteria that causes acne.

- Decreases swelling, redness, and inflammation.

- Stimulates white blood cells involved in the immune system.

Infrared LED If you have been paying attention, you know that infrared (IR) waves are invisible. Therefore, if you have a device made with infrared LEDs, how the hell do you know when it's on? Hopefully you bought it from a clever manufacturer that either, 1) mixed it with other visible LEDs like red or amber or, 2) they built in a lighted control switch indicating when the device is actually turned on. IR LEDs can penetrate the skin between 5-10mm deep. They have been used to treat ulcers and wounds and have even been shown to treat cellulite! [174][175] IR LED generates warmth and can relax tight muscles, increase circulation, and help products penetrate deeper into the skin. For all the aforementioned reasons, this LED is commonly used in pain relief devices that are good for sore backs or achy joints. If all else fails, we guess you can sit on it and run your own cellulite reduction experiment. Let us know how that goes; we are sure you will. Behold the benefits of infrared LED:

- Generates warmth, relaxing muscles and encouraging product penetration.

- Helps heal ulcers and wounds.

- Can bring relief to achy, sore body parts.

Combined LED Therapy We know you are already heady with excitement about the anti-aging, acne clearing, and pain reducing potential for LEDs. The only thing more riveting than the ever-increasing database of positive results associated with their use would be the types of results expected when *different* LEDs are combined in the same device to deliver a myriad of benefits to the user. We know! The possibilities are mind bending. And yes, there is more delightful data to support the use of multiple wavelengths simultaneously directed at the skin, delivering even more powerful results. Treatment with four colors: amber, light red, red and infrared significantly increased the number of viable fibroblasts and type I collagen expression. Also, the combinations of amber with infrared, and light red with red, led to better anti- photoaging outcomes than single LED wavelengths[176].

We are also seeing combinations such as blue and red to zap zits and concurrently promote healing of those zits. **LightStim**®-is our favorite LED manufacturer because they are at the forefront of combined LED technology with their MultiWave® Patent. They have three wands, each combining the best LEDs to get the job done: LightStim® for Wrinkles, LightStim® for Acne and LightStim® for Pain. Their products are made right here in the USA in Irvine, California, and they have a 90-day money-back guarantee. The family is amazing and stand behind their products. Sure, you can buy a less expensive (non-returnable) device on eBay from Taiwan, but you will not be supporting a local business using quality, patented technology.

IPL Intense pulsed light (IPL) treatments are often referred to as photo-facials. IPL utilizes the same wavelengths of light as LED, but they are very different. LEDs generate scattered light, like an ordinary light bulb. It is cool, light and non-ablative (that means it won't tear apart your tissue). To give you an example of opposite land light, lasers use focused light in one wavelength (visualize a laser beam glowing in one color, like Darth Vader's lightsaber in red or Yoda's in green). These target one specific problem or use. This light can be very hot and some can cut through tissue like a knife through butter. We are not discussing lasers in this book because, 1) there are a million lasers on the market, each with their own unique function and, 2) in most states, estheticians are not licensed to use lasers (that includes lasers to remove hair). A medical doctor well versed in lasers and their use would be the one to answer your questions.

So then, what is IPL? It's somewhere in between LEDs and lasers. Similar to LEDs, IPL uses scattered light, and it is non-ablative. Similar to lasers, IPL generates heat and it also puts out a lot of energy. But because IPL is using many wavelengths of light at once, it can treat different conditions. If a technician wanted to zero in on treating a specific problem, she could use a filter to allow only certain wavelengths to reach the skin. The specific light energy is directed towards specific chemical targets in the skin called chromophores. Examples of chromophore targets in the skin are:

- melanin (the pigment in skin or hair)

- blood (specifically oxyhemoglobin – a hemoglobin molecule carrying an oxygen which turns red)

- tattoo ink

The chromophore target attracts the light and heat from the IPL. It attracts so much light and heat that the unwanted hyperpigmentation, hair, capillary, or tattoo is destroyed. The body just absorbs the debris and heals. If you have ever had hair removal using light, you can actually feel a pop when the hair blows up. No, this does not feel good, especially in the bikini area, so you better down a few Advil® before hitting the clinic. So, to be clear, both lasers and IPL can do some of the same things, like remove unwanted hair, so ask a lot of questions when seeking out light treatments. You want to be certain about which modality you will be receiving and who will be the licensed technician delivering said treatment. Each state has their own regulations about who can operate IPL and laser machines, and most of those rulings are still murky, so check out your local laws and then find someone who is licensed *and* very experienced.

What type of skin is eligible for IPL? Did you ever wonder why there are so many white cars in Arizona? Autotrader wanted to know too, so they put two cars out in the scorching sun, one black and one white. The interior of the black car reached 130 °F while the interior of the white car only rose to 113°F. That is because the color black attracts more light, and therefore, more heat. Same thing goes with the skin. Darker tissue with more melanin will attract more light and heat from IPL. If you want to use IPL to reduce a spot of hyperpigmentation, it is best if the spot is dark and the surrounding skin is very light. The IPL will be absorbed by the dark spot, giving it a little sizzle, while the surrounding tissue stays cool. The spot will scab up, fall off, and will usually be lighter after healing. You can imagine how this will not work so well, and could even be disastrous, if the surrounding epidermis was also dark and absorbed a significant amount of light and heat. There could be a lot more fizzle-bo-bizzle going on than just your brown blotch.

People with lighter skin tones (Fitzpatrick Skin Types 1-3) with a dark spot (in fact, the darker the better) are ideal candidates for treatment with IPL. The more contrast between the base color and target color, the better. People with darker skin tones (Fitzpatrick Skin Types 4-6) are not good candidates for IPL (and laser). As previously explained, the highly pigmented skin surrounding the problem area can attract the light and the heat and be injured, leaving the skin darker (hyperpigmented) or lighter (hypopigmented) than it was before. Same goes for hair removal; the lighter the skin and the darker the hair, the better the outcome. Keep in mind that if you are thinking of getting some pesky hairs zapped, get it done *before* they turn white... after that, you'll have to turn to the tweezer.

Who's Your Tech? The technician needs to be able to determine your Fitzpatrick Skin Type to assess whether IPL can work for you.

Since we are more racially diverse than ever and some of us have mixed ethnicities, it takes a professional with a lot of experience asking the right questions to determine one's candidacy. Let's say you have a combo of white and black ancestors. Even if your skin looks fair, it may respond to light like a darker tissue tone. An experienced technician will take a thorough skin history, identify potential risks and avoid any chance of injury.

Ultrasonic An esthetician walks into a bar... oh you know this is going to be good... it was actually us making a run into our local wine bar while working on this book. As much as it may seem like it, we were *not* writing under the influence, but we were having some WI-FI frustrations that day. We threw in the towel, jumped on our bikes, and headed over to our friend's wine shop to keep working. Little did we know that sitting in a corner would be a coterie of cosmetologists being mesmerized by a small, silver, vibrating, warming electrical device. Now, we know what ya'll are thinking because we were thinking the same thing and imagined that perhaps one of these new-agey, at-home, sex toy parties had been uprooted and moved to the local wine shop. But regardless, we were determined to find out more and forwent eavesdropping. We walked right up to the table and asked, "What the hell is that?" And thus began our journey into the land of ultrasonic facials.

You may already be familiar with ultrasonic waves if you have ever had an ultrasound, which we happen to think is the coolest technology on the planet! Let's face it, you can see right the f*ck into your body! Think about this for just one second... and then think what life was like *before* we had this technology. Want to know what that pain radiating from your left ovary is? Cut your body open. What's that lump in your neck? Cut your body open. Brain tumor... ok you get the picture, pun intended. Ultrasonic waves can take a selfie of your unborn baby, your uterine fibroid, and can help direct an orthopedic surgeon's needle as she injects a shoulder with cortisone. Ultrasonic waves are actually sound waves that humans cannot hear. During an ultrasound, these waves transmit through the body and bounce back when they contact tissue, creating an image of what's inside.

Another cool use is that a lower intensity of these sound waves can be used to clean things. Tanis remembers that in a microbiology lab where she used to work, there was a little fluid-filled chamber with a tray. They put instruments that needed to be cleaned onto the tray, flipped the switch, and essentially, the ultrasonic waves would shake the shit right off of the instruments. She quickly figured out that it was also fabulous for cleaning her jewelry and glasses. Then, she saw ultrasonic in action again while working at a hospital. She had noticed that the nurses were using a little device to help topical medications penetrate into the patient's skin, sans needles! Indeed, these sound waves assist in transdermal drug delivery, often referred to as sonophoresis, and research continues to identify more molecules that can be nudged through the stratum corneum using this technology. [177] Hmmm... cleaning... product penetration... well you can guess why it wasn't long before an ultrasonic device ended up on the beauty scene and in the hands of some wine swilling cosmetologists.

The exact device they were fiddling with that day was the **ZOE**® **by QYKSonic**®. It vibrates, and it warms while it assists penetration. We know, what's a girl not to love? And speaking of love, guess what we stumbled upon at the last skin convention? QYKSonic® put the puzzle pieces together and came up with a device called the **ZOE**® that cleans *and* assists with product penetration! It is adorable, durable, colorful, made of medical grade silicon, has no disposable pieces or attachments and is a breeze to clean. The ZOE® not only delivers over 6,000 pulsations per minute, but each side has different sized bristles specifically designed for either removing grime, makeup and oil or for pulsing product down deep. You can use it 300 times before it needs recharging, so it just became our new favorite travel buddy.

We also think it's cuter and way more hypoallergenic than a purse dog, so move over Mr. Amazing, you'll find a ZOE® snuggled in the bottom of our bags!

WHAT YOUR ESTHETICIAN
REALLY WANTED TO TELL YOU

- Before you go high tech, go classic and regularly get traditional facials. Make it the foundation of your beauty routine.

- Get an LED device and light your way to better skin. Choose the device for your skin care goals and then actually use it!

- IPL can be used to eradicate brown blotches, unwanted hair, capillaries, and tattoos. Make sure your technician is licensed and delves deeply into your ethnicity to determine your Fitzpatrick rating and the treatment that is appropriate for you.

- Ultrasonic is used to cleanse and help your products deeply penetrate. This is the Barry White of skincare devices; it's our first, our last, our everything.

COVID-19

skin care

21

COVID-19 SKIN CARE

WE ALL WEAR MASKS

This book had 20 chapters. We wish it still did. And we wish that none of our loved ones, no strangers, or even our "enemies" will have to suffer from the direct and not so direct devastating effects of COVID-19, the first pandemic since 1918. We send out a big healing virtual hug to our sister esties, our clients, family, friends. Damn, we send it out to the whole world and pray that the contents of this chapter rapidly become obsolete. Until then, read on for tips about how to address the emerging skin conditions related to the new precautionary measures that we are taking to reduce our risk of contracting coronavirus.

Neddy's Take:

Just like that, it happened. As the first cases of coronavirus in the United States were tracked and reported on, the news broadcast the closure of all non-essential businesses seemingly overnight. Rumors and facts swirled, warning us that law enforcement may come to ensure doors to businesses classified as such were locked and stayed locked, just in case anyone dared to rebel.

My salon suite was shuttered with no reopening date on the horizon. I still remember it so vividly, the image of my beloved suite, full of cherry-picked top-of-the-line organic products, stacks of freshly laundered linens, and dreams of helping thousands of clients tackle their most troublesome skin challenges. As my key clicked in the lock of my little treatment room, I pondered if I would ever be allowed to return and use that key again. I felt my business slipping through my hands, the hands that had so lovingly cared for my clients, many of whom had become friends and confidants. In an instant, my beloved business had turned upside down, and my life as I had known it up until that moment would never be the same.

I think most estheticians would agree COVID-19 has been the biggest threat to our profession and challenge to our industry than anything else we have ever faced. And our tribe has been through a lot. Here's a few of the most recent challenges we have overcome:

- The 2008 economic crash.

- Enhanced educational requirements and the adjustment of laws as HIV became a household word.

- The 2019 regulation banning esties from being hired as contractors eliminating thousands of jobs.

- The advent of Amazon created a marked decrease in spa retail sales (and our income) as online purchases of skincare products exploded.

But these all seemed to pale in comparison to the closure of spas around the world for fear of spreading a highly contagious and deadly disease.

When my livelihood was abruptly halted, I suddenly found myself unemployed. Wondering if it would ever be safe to return to life as I knew it BC (Before COVID), I found myself feeling guarded and cautious about divulging my professional knowledge of skincare. I became paranoid and anxious and started thinking that if I share all these skin care tips and tricks, and everybody can buy anything they want online (including illegal professional strength products), who's ever going to want to come back to me? People won't **need** me anymore. I will become obsolete, a profession of the past. And in an ironic turn of events like in a horror film, I would have to become an Amazon truck driver delivering the same products I told millions of people about in this book ultimately putting me out of business... forever!! No!!! This was a nightmare I direly wanted to prevent.

Our pandemic introduced us to an *Era of Uncertainty*, stoking self-doubt in all of us, and I was suffering from a severe case of the wobbles. It's easy to fall into the trap of "withholding knowledge" out of fear of not having a business to return to if you give away all the wisdom for free.

However, when I decided to become an esthetician, I truly wanted to help other people. Being able to be of service to others has always been my WHY. And I have learned that in the face of adversity, one must always strip themselves down to their WHY. It's the impetus to clarity and the jump start to creativity. Hoarding information out of fear of loss is the biggest disservice any professional can do to themselves, and ultimately to others who stand to benefit from their expertise.

I realized early on that despite any fear or anxiety I was feeling, I would not let it stop me from being of service as I had always been. Now more than ever, estheticians need to help their clients in every way possible regardless of monetary compensation. Being an esthetician is so much more than the facials we perform and the products we prescribe. People choose to trust us with the care of their skin; their face. In us, they find relief, confidence, and nurturing because they trust we have their best interest at heart. I'd created intimate bonds with my clients, and no pandemic was going to stop me from being there for them because it's an honor to have had them as clients in the first place.

I shook off my fear and leaped into action. I sent out email updates to my clients regularly, offered virtual consultations, and customized DIY facial boxes with personalized instructions. I implemented new and creative ways to keep engaged with my clients on social media via skin tip videos and educational content posts. Of course, Tanis and I pushed forward with the completion of this book with the addition of one more special chapter.

And the response? A touching reply from my clients welcoming, supporting, and encouraging my efforts. The universe has such a lovely way of giving back in immeasurable and unexpected ways. During my struggle, my clients would be the ones to save my business with an outpouring of warmth, love, and grace. All because I chose to let my WHY be stronger than the storm that threatened it. I continued to give, and my clients gave back. My business and I have changed, for the better, as I found unique ways to help my clients help themselves when I couldn't physically be there for them. And I know that when it's safe, they will return to my little treatment room, where I can once again work my magic. I can hear that key clicking already!

The "Maskne" Phenomenon

Hats off to the frontline workers, surgeons, forensic scientists, perfusionists, anesthesiologists, fighter pilots, beer brewers and the myriad of professionals that have been wearing masks BC (Before COVID) and are now thinking "What's the fuss people? Put on your freaking masks." We now understand your plight and appreciate your dedication to your job and the very special PPE that you must wear to do it. Perhaps you have already suffered in silence with some of the strange things that our skin is doing since the masses have had to gown up to go out. So, finally, we're happy to announce, the "Esties are to the Rescue" with remedies to this new set of skin ailments. We would have piped in sooner if we had been clued in to the deleterious side effects of masking up, but alas, late is better than never to this mask-querade. Let's do this people. Let's tackle Maskne.

Maskne [**mask**-nee] : *Maskne* is acne or other skin irritation that results from wearing a mask, especially a medical, N95, or cloth face mask.

Ok people, don't act so mystified here. Remember when you were charging through the house as a child (or possibly more recently avec martini glass in hand) and you slipped on your (choose one according to your generation) 1) Lincoln Log, 2) Weeble, 3) Transformer, 4) Tamagotchi or 5) Kung Zhu, and went carpet surfing through the family room on your shins? Congrats, you just earned yourself a royal treatment rug burn that will go down in history and forever leave strange white tracks on your knees that never seem to tan. Alas, welcome to the wacky world of mask wearing. All this scratching and a tugging while we are trying to run away at the mouth is causing some serious fabric-to-skin abrasion, just like your rug rubbed shanks, and that, my friends, needs some serious TLC.

So, what's going on inside that viral curtain that's creating a pimple pandemonium? Maskne is basically acne mechanica, a type of breakout caused by friction, heat, and occlusion on the skin. Combine this with a jungle-like environment created by moisture trapped under the mask generated by talking, breathing, and sweating and you've got yourself the perfect situation for clogged pores and the proliferation of *P. Acnes* along with a multitude of other bacteria, yeast, and mold. The skin can also become dry, itchy, and like most of the veggies, we eat… raw. Other mask-induced COVID conundrums include:

Folliculitus This is when bacteria and yeast infect hair follicles causing them to become red, irritated, and filled with pus. Oh joy.

Rosacea Exacerbated by heat and stress, add masks to the list of things that can induce flare-ups.

Contact Dermatitis Irritation caused by rubbing along with formaldehyde and bronopol found in surgical masks can trigger allergic responses leading to redness, swelling, and even blistering of the skin.

Seborrheic Dermatitis Pissed off sebaceous glands can get nasty, forming scaly, dandruff-like patches that flake and itch.

Maskne Prevention

An ounce of prevention is worth a pound of cure. So, follow these easy guidelines to help ward off unnecessary mask-related skin complications:

- **Wash Your F*cking Mask** We know, we know. We throw them in the bottom of our not-so-immaculate purse, in our car console, on our dashboard, yes, on the floor of our car. We breathe in them, sneeze in them, cough in them. Our lipstick lines the interior and our noses go foundation-free as it all coats the inside of our mask. Bad bacteria harboring in the mask will co-mingle with the good bacteria that make up the protective microbiome of your skin. This creates disruption in the balance of your skin, making it more susceptible to a bombardment of bad bacteria and breakouts. So, honestly people - put a little more effort into giving your masks a ride in the wishy-washy and clean up your routine. Skip detergents with fragrance and especially brighteners that often include diatomaceous earth which can be irritating. And while you're skipping out, avoid fabric softeners, too.

- **Wash Your F*cking Face** See a trend here? We wrote a whole chapter on this facial essential but just in case you've already forgotten, your face is filthy and harbors millions of microbes. Wash it before donning your mask and after long periods of wear.

- **Shelve the Makeup** This is your opportunity to forget the foundation and give your skin a much-needed break from MAC attacks. Get your glam on by reinventing your eye makeup and lashes. Colored mascara, anyone?

- **Quench Parched Skin** Wearing a lotion rich with Ceramides and Hyaluronic Acid will help hold moisture in the skin while enhancing its barrier function. Dimethicone will help provide glide so that friction and irritation from your mask is reduced.

And like any new skin care product, get ready to try a little experimentation to find the formulation, viscosity, and finish that's right for you. We highly recommend the **Sleep It Off Slumber Mask by NUÅGE9®**, formulated to calm and soothe during twinkle time. Backed by clinical testing, Syricalm® is naturally soothing herbal extracts that help to reduce redness, inflammation, and irritation. Pentavitin® is a natural saccharide that hydrates for up to 72 hours while Ceramides support the recovery and maintenance of the skin's protective barrier. Crafted with a potent blend of Hyaluronic Acid, this product moisturizes through multiple layers of the skin. Say "lights out" to fine lines, irritability, and flakiness. And please, remember your hands! Excess washing and sanitization can leave them dry and cracked.

- **Banish Breakouts** This book is jam-packed full of pimple popping advice we recommend to force breakouts into submission. But in addition, maskne skin needs a little more TLC than just your run-of-the-mill flare-up. Again, NUÅGE9® to the rescue with their **Blue Mist Corrective Tonique**. Spray away irritation and breakouts with a blend of botanicals targeted to calm and heal mask-induced skin challenges. Blue Tansy helps to clear congested pores and reduce redness while Mallow calms over-sensitized skin. Backed by clinical testing, Poria Mushroom and Reed Grass effectively reduce inflammation and strongly support skin in dealing with external stressors. Insider Tip: Spray on the inside of your mask to freshen it up throughout the day!

Tanis' & Neddy's Sidebar: Mask Face Off

Are Cloth Masks Superior to Disposable Masks?

Neddy ⚞ Tanis ⚟

An N95 mask is actually the winner here, but these masks are reserved for our fearless frontline workers. The best homemade cloth masks actually achieved better filtration (79 percent) than surgical masks (62 percent to 65 percent) in a peer-reviewed study at the Wake Forest Institute of Regenerative Medicine. Cloth masks are also re-usable and come in a variety of patterns and colors. Satin masks create less friction and may offer less irritation than other masks, but they hold in heat. They are also not as breathable as cotton or disposables. Cotton is more breathable, but it harbors more bacteria than other materials, making them a sanctuary for bad bacteria. If this is your mask of choice, frequently wash it. Silk provides lots of glide, keeps moisture in the skin, and doesn't tend to be a major crash pad for microbes. But again, this material needs to see the inside of your washing machine on a daily basis.

COVID-19 Skin Side Effects

And in the beginning... the only strong indicators that one had COVID were coughing, shortness of breath, and a fever. But as we moved into the late spring and early summer of 2020, everything from loss of taste and smell, to hallucinations, to a chicken pox like rash and even "COVID toes" were clues that the coronavirus may have invaded your personal space. In fact, Tanis had just self-quarantined in March 2020 when her skin erupted in what she thought was an untimely breakout of adult chicken pox and a case of the runs that turned the toilet paper shortage into a major first world problem. The symptoms persisted for over a month and something kept her in isolation, even though no-one at that time was talking about those particular symptoms being related to that nasty virus. And a few months later... skin rashes make the 5 o'clock news along with toes that are looking like someone went to Napa and did some serious grape stomping. Yes, the coronavirus had an effect on some people's skin with few remedies available except for some over-the-counter treatments like cortisone, calamine lotion, or a bit of Neosporin applied to angry blisters. Alas, these skin ailments recede on their own, with little to be done to accelerate the process. Patience is indeed virtuous at this point, as it has been for any symptoms related to COVID-19.

And this particular potential repercussion wasn't noted until about six to nine months after people had coronavirus... hair loss. Researchers say that the hair loss some are experiencing is consistent with a condition called Telogen Effluvium (TE). Hair falling out in large clumps while brushing or washing it is a clue you may be experiencing TE. So far, people who have had severe cases of COVID are most likely to experience balding. But the link to stress associated with not just catching the virus but trying to hold our shit together during a pandemic is *real* and can also trigger TE.

If you are experiencing significant hair loss, you may want to talk with your doc about possible solutions. We immediately thought of Latisse® that functions by keeping hair in the growth phase, preventing it from entering the telogen phase. The generic name of Latisse® is bimatoprost, and yes, it works, but regulating agencies are slow at the wheel to put their stamp of approval on any new applications for a drug. Allergan has studies underway to demonstrate its effectiveness on the scalp and eyebrows (which we already know because that's how we grew our brows back). Hurry people... we would like to stick our entire heads in that stuff because we got some braiding to do.

The DIY Estie Phenomenon

We know, after all the sage advice in this book, you went out and found yourself an amazing, caring, intelligent estie (who has also read this book) and you've been going steady for a few months now. Enter the Black Swan: COVID-19 and you had to "stop seeing each other as much" and suddenly "needed your own space" for a while. Well, we know you didn't want to cheat on your estie bestie. So instead, you've decided to opt in for some self-gratification. A little "alone time" and

you're looking in the mirror thinking, "It really can't be that hard….
can it? A little micro here, a little peel there, jab some zits with a pin and
I'm good." Or… are you being very, very bad? Here's the scoop with a
sprinkle of encouragement and a good dash of caution to all the DIY
Esties out there. Take heed.

Microdermabrasion When this procedure was first introduced,
the equipment was large, and heavy, and cost more than our first car.
Only spas could afford the space and money of said equipment. But
like computers, microdermabrasion machines kept getting smaller, and
cheaper, and well, frankly, better.

We both own a "DIY" hand held microderm machine and we can
dig it. Even with a great piece of equipment, it is still best to have your
esthetician perform this treatment because it can be tricky to evenly and
consistently move the wand over the surface of the skin. And uneven
application equals uneven results. If possible, have your estie bestie
perform this procedure.

Chemical Peels We wish there was an easy way to advise on peels.
Something simple like "Anything under (fill in the blank) % is safe to use
on all skin types"! To an extent, this is true. Anything you find in the
drugstore, Ulta Beauty, or Sephora is probably safe for most skins. But
beyond that, buyers beware! We saw some shit for sale on the internet
that could kill people, yes, kill! Concentrated salicylic acid solutions
strong enough to put people into intoxication (and we don't mean the
fun kind brought on by partaking of Absinthe). For the gory deets, go
read chapter 19. On that note, just say no to DIY chemical peels. We've
seen "Peels Gone Wild" season 1, and it's not worth a repeat.

LED This one, gets two snaps up in a circle! As a matter of fact, if you
do not have a home-use LED you are using almost every day, then it's
not going to work optimally. Using LED is like going to the gym; once a
month is not going to show lasting visible results. And if your esthetician
has been selling you on this treatment, sure it's nice for a "cherry on
top" glow, or for an immediate reduction in swelling from extractions.
But an estie that's a keeper will sell you an LED wand to take home.

Laser Hair Removal First of all, it's probably not a real laser, and if it is an actual laser, not only is it illegal but we highly recommend that you best not be putting that anywhere near your eyes, or your cooch… or any part of your body for that matter. We've seen burns that left people's skin looking like this season's trending leopard print. Most at-home devices use intense pulse light (IPL) technology as the method of hair removal.

How does IPL remove hair? The dark hair absorbs controlled flashes of light in the follicles lying below the skin's surface. The absorbed light heats the dark hair, making it, well, explode. This damages the follicle, making it difficult or impossible for it to produce another hair. If done right (key word), it does not damage the surrounding tissue. However, IPL does *not* permanently remove all hair. At best, it can reduce the total number of body hairs if done correctly.

Here's another tidbit to consider: darlings, at-home devices might likely have limited battery power, so the consistent intensity of your pulsating light will be compromised, giving you underwhelming results and buyer's remorse.

Lastly, these devices are not "one size fits all". Think of IPL (and lasers) like the mean girls in high school that don't let just anyone sit at their table. IPL technology is "not inclusive" and prefers dark hair nestled in pale skin. That is because it should zero in on pigments in the hair follicle (and not in our skin) so the contrast between skin and hair is necessary to be effective and safe. People with pale skin and dark hair are "included" in this clique and are the ideal candidates. Everyone else is zapping their cash away and potentially zapping their skin.

Dermaplaning This procedure of hair removal in conjunction with exfoliation sounds familiar, right? Maybe it's something that you used to watch your daddy do every morning in the bathroom mirror or that you still dread before donning your favorite skirt. Yes, dermaplaning is this century's ultimate version of razor use on the skin and can be compared to "shaving on crack". With that being said, we have seen a wide range of how this can be performed and just as wide a range of laws governing this procedure.

In the doctor's office, this is what it looks like: a sterile blade is positioned at a 45-degree angle and glided slowly across your skin removing dead cells, (possibly) scar tissue, and other debris that makes the skin's surface look uneven.

At home, this is what it looks like: the Bare By Schick™ Dermaplaning Wand that's designed with clever ergonomics keeping the blade at the correct angle. Basically, a safety razor designed to remove hair and any extra skin cells hanging out on the surface of the face. Do not expect to get the same results as a scalpel in the hands of an expertly trained doc (or in some states, a nurse or an esthetician, depending on the laws). Do expect an inexpensive and safe way to smooth out skin. And then… there's always your daddy's Mach3.

And in our last attempt to crush an urban myth once and for all, no, shaving does not make your hair grow in darker or thicker. How could shaving change your genetics? Our hair dye is def not making our hair grow in less gray, think people, think! The reason this mythology continues to circulate is probably based on these facts: 1) When you shave, the hair is cut blunt so when it first emerges from your skin, it can feel more "pokey" (and thicker?) than it normally does as that erect sharp end sticks straight outta your face. After some time, the tip will soften, the hair will bend downward, and that flaccid follicle will feel like it used to. 2) When new hair makes its debut, it has not been exposed to any light and will appear darker than it normally does. Again, if you give it some sunshine and let it grow out completely, it can appear lighter over time.

Microneedling Also known as collagen induction, this procedure involves using a device with small, short needles to poke the skin, triggering it to repair itself… meanwhile making more collagen and elastin. Again, laws vary from state to state on the legality of this procedure as performed by an esthetician. Doctors can perform this treatment and, in some situations, it is possible for a person working in a medically supervised clinic to perform it, as well. So, even though it may not be legal for an estie to microneedle you, no one can prevent you from sticking needles in your own face. Microneedling devices can be purchased with sterile needles, but after the first use, they are no longer microbe free and you will have to consider ways to sanitize your device. And similar to microdermabrasion, you are striving for an even application of the device across the skin. We can tell you that this is easier said than done, as we have made several lame attempts to microneedle ourselves. Reason being? Those little pricks hurt like heck and we simply could not complete the task on our own.

DIY Takeaway

We say, let your DIY estie flag fly free… with caution, and even better, with guidance. During COVID-times, Neddy offered mini "Awaken SOS" boxes. They have definitely come to the rescue of many skincare SOS emergencies. With customizable options, step-by-step instructions, and sage advice from a professional estie who cares, your DIY facials will be far from mediocre. From virtual spa parties to self-care nights at home, these mail-order kits were a no-brainer. For more amazing products that are formulated by esties for serious at-home care, check out the NUÅGE9® line at the **Ask The Estheticians Shop**.

WHAT YOUR ESTHETICIAN **REALLY** WANTED TO TELL YOU

- Maskne is real but you can lessen its effects by choosing the right mask and practicing proper hygiene.

- There are other mask-induced skin quandaries, such as folliculitis, rosacea, and dermatitis. Beware of the symptoms and seek help from a professional if problems persist.

- COVID time is DIY time. But it doesn't mean you can stop listening to your estie. Follow professional advice on how to care for your skin at home and know when to say "no".

- A plethora of products are being produced, especially for ailments related to mask wearing and hand washing. Seek out products designed to address specific problems and check out specialty products made by NUÅGE9® for what ails you.

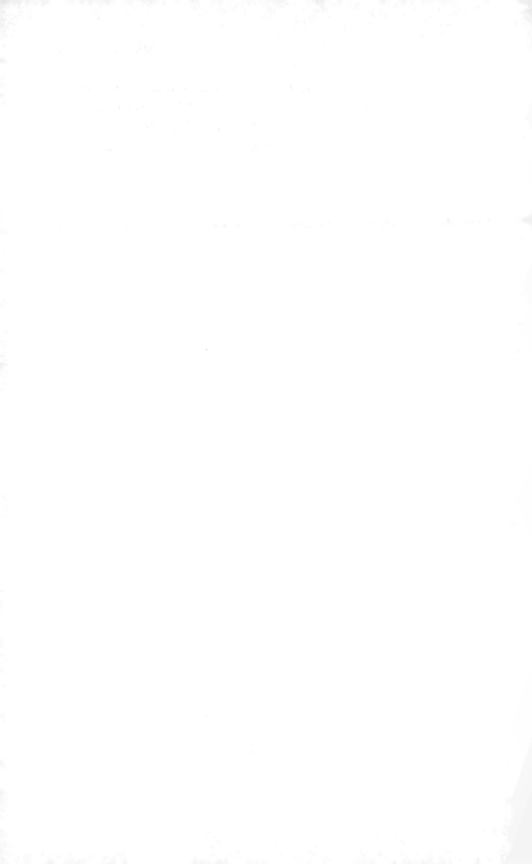

AFTERWORD

Holy Crap! It's the ending and you may be wondering where, exactly, do you begin? First, there's an index for this book; use it to help you re-locate all the topics that are hot for you. Second, get an esthetician. If you already have one, we congratulate you and encourage you to verbally give that person permission to tell you the good, the bad, and the ugly truth about your skin. Remember that you are a team… and then take their f*cking advice, question them, try their products and show up for your appointments. You will die prettier doing so. If you are an esthetician, we hope this book has inspired you to put on your big girl chonies and stop withholding information from your clients because you are lazy, clueless, greedy, or scared. Energize yourself, educate yourself, elevate yourself, and then share.

And of course, this is not the end of our romance with the epidermis. The skin industry changes faster than iPhone versions and we are always on the prowl for superlative products and tantalizing trends. We can stay in touch at www.asktheestheticians.com where you can actually, well, ask your burning questions about beauty. We'd love to chat. You can also join us on Facebook, Instagram and Twitter, where we banter, ponder and pontificate about the crazy shit we see in this industry. We'd love for you to come get crazy with us. Even better, let's go cuckoo in person, we're always hanging around skin conventions and spas and would love to meet you. We post our whereabouts on social media, at least when we want to be found.

We hope you did not leave a page of this book unturned, as there are juicy tidbits scattered throughout… even in the chapters that you may think are meh or not for you. And remember, if you've got questions, never be afraid to ASK. We wrote this book because… someone did!

WORKS CITED

1. **DeNoon, Daniel J.** WebMD Parenting News. *WebMD.* [Online] September 14, 2011. www.webmd.com/parenting/news/20110914/parents-kids-doctors-balk-at-talk-about-weight#1.

2. *A population based study of acne and body mass index in adolescents.* **Halvorsen, J A, et al.** 1, January 2012, Arch Dermatol, Vol. 148, pp. 131-132.

3. *Diet and acne update: carbohydrates emerge as the main culprit.* **Mahmood SN, Bowe WP.** April 2014, J Drugs Dermatol, Vol. 13(4), pp. 428-435.

4. *Acne vulgaris: a disease of Western civilization.* **Cordain, L.** 12, December 2002, Arch Dermatol, Vol. 138, pp. 1584-1590.

5. *Milk consumption and acne in adolescent girls.* **Adebamowo, C A, et al.** 4, May 40, 2006, Dermatol Online J, Vol. 12, p. 1.

6. *Family history, body mass index, selected dietary factors, menstrual history, and risk of moderate to severe acne in adolescents and young adults.* **Di Landro, A.** 6, December 2012, J Am Acad Dermatol, Vol. 67, pp. 1129-1135.

7. *Milk consumption and acne in teenage boys.* **Adebamowo, C A, et al.** 5, May 2008, J Am Acad Dermatol, Vol. 58, pp. 787-793.

8. *Dietary changes favorably affect bone remodeling in older adults.* **Heaney, R P, et al.** 10, October 1999, Vol. 99, pp. 1228-1233.

9. *Prospective study of colorectal cancer risk in men and plasma levels of insulin-like growth factor (IGF)-I and IGF-binding protein-3.* **Ma, J, et al.** 1999, J Natl Cancer Inst, Vol. 91, pp. 620-625.

10. *Effects of neonatal flutamide treatment on hippocampal neurogenesis and synaptogenesis correlate with depression-like behaviors in preadolescent male rats.* **Zhang, J T, et al.** 1, 2010, Neuroscience, Vol. 169, pp. 544-554.

11. *Testosterone and social isolation influence adult neurogenesis in the denate gyrus of male rats.* **Spritzer, MD, et al.** 2011, Neuroscience, Vol. 195, pp. 180-190.

12. *Androgen physiology.* **Davison, S L and Bell, R.** 2, 2006, Semin Reprod Med, Vol. 24, pp. 71-77.

13. *The sexually dimorphic role of androgens in human metabolic disease.* **Schiffer, L, et al.** 3, 2017, Eur J Endocrinol, Vol. 177, pp. R125-R143.

14. *Quantitative documentation of a premenstrual flare of facial acne in adult women.* **Lucky, A.W.** April 2004, Arch Dermatol, Vol. 140(4), pp. 423-424.

15. *Increasing Benzodiazepine Prescriptions and Overdose Mortality in the United States, 1996-2013.* **Bachhuber, M A, et al.** 4, 2016, Am J Public Health, Vol. 106, pp. 686-688.

16. *A specific breeding problem of sheep on subterranean clover pastures in Western Australia.* **Bennetts, H W, Underwood, E J and Shier, F L.** 1946, Australian Veterinary Journal, Vol. 22, pp. 2-12.

17. *Molecular aspects of phytoestrogen selective binding at estrogen receptors.* **Turner, J V, Agatonovic-Kustrin, S and Glass, B D.** 8, August 2007, Journal of Pharmaceutical Sciences, Vol. 96, pp. 1879-1885.

18. **Johnson, I and Williamson, Gary.** *Phytochemical Functional Foods.* Boca Raton: CRC Press, 2003. pp. 66-68.

19. *Phytochemical mimicry of reproductive hormones and modulation of herbivore fertility by phytoestrogens.* **Hughes, C L.** 1988, Environmental Health Perspectives, Vol. 78, pp. 171-174.

20. *The potential health effects of dietary phytoestrogens.* **Rietjens, I M, Louisse, J and Beekman, K.** 11, June 2017, British Journal of Pharmacology, Vol. 174, pp. 1263-1280.

21. *Sex hormones and skin collagen content in postmenopausal women.* **Brincat, M, et al.** 6402, 1983, Br Med J (Clin Res Ed), Vol. 287, pp. 1337-1338.

22. **Korach, K S.** *Reproductive and Developmental Toxicology.* New York City: Marcel Dekker Ltd., 1998. pp. 278-279.

23. *Estrogen-like endocrine disrupting chemicals affecting puberty in humans-a review.* **Roy, J R, Chakraborty, S and Chakraborty, T R.** 6, June 2009, Med Sci Monit, Vol. 15, pp. RA 137-145.

24. *An extensive new literature concerning low-dose effects of bisphenol A shows the need for a new risk assessment.* **Vom Saal, F S and Hughes, C.** 8, August 2005, Environmental Health Perspectives, Vol. 113, pp. 926-933

25. *Phthalates and other additives in plastics: human exposure and associated health outcomes.* **Meeker, J D, Sathyanarayana, S and Swan, S H.** 1526, July 2009, Philosophical Transactions of the Roral Society B, Vol. 364, pp. 2097-2113.

26. **World Health Organization.** Dioxins and their effects on human health. *World Health Organization.* [Online] October 4, 2016. http://www.who.int/news-room/fact-sheets/detail/dioxins-and-their-effects-on-human-health.

27. *A novel effect of dioxin: exposure during pregnancy severely impairs mammary gland differentiation.* **Vorderstrasse, B A, et al.** 2004, Toxicol Sci, Vol. 78, pp. 248-257.

28. *Cancer risk assessment using blood dioxin levels and daily dietary TEQ intake in general populations of industrial and non-industrial countries.* **Schechter, A and Olson, J R.** 5-7, Mar-April 1997, Chemosphere, Vol. 34, pp. 1569-1577.

29. *Essential plant oils and headache mechanisms.* **Gobel, H, et al.** 2, Oct 1995, Phytomedicine, Vol. 2, pp. 93-102.

30. *Inhalation of Odorants for Weight Reduction.* **Hirsch, A R and Gomez, R.** 2, August 1994, The International Journal of Obesity, Vol. 18, p. 79.

31. **Parker-Pope, Tara.** The Hormone Decision. New York: Pocket Books, 2008.

32. *Highly abundant defense proteins in human sweat as revealed by targeted proteomics and label-free quantification mass spectrometry.* **Csosz, E, et al.** 10, 2015, J Eur Acad Dermatol Venereol, Vol. 29, pp. 2024-2031.

33. *Influence of the pH-value on the growth of Staphylococcus epidermis. Staphylococcus aureus, and Propionibacteriem acnes in continuous culture.* **Korting, H C, et al.** 1, 1992, Zentralbl Hyg Umweltmed, Vol. 193, pp. 78-90.

34. *Reduced expression of dermcidin, a peptide active against propionibacterium acnes, in sweat of patients with acne vulgaris.* **Nakano, T, et al.** 7, 2015, Acta Derm Venereol, Vol. 95, pp. 783-786.

35. *Effect of regular sauna on epidermal barrier function and stratum corneum water-holding capacity in vivo in humans: a controlled study.* **Kowatzki, D, et al.** 2, 2008, Dermatology, Vol. 217, pp. 173-180.

36. *Human elimination of phthalate compounds: blood, urine, and sweat (BUS) study.* **Genuis, S J, et al.** 2012, Scientific World Journal, Vol. 2012, p. 615068.

37. *Arsenic, cadmium lead, and mercury in sweat: a systematic review.* **Sears, M E, Kerr, K J and Bray, R I.** 2012, J Environ Public Health, Vol. 2012, p. 184745.

38. **Diet Health Club.** How many calories are burned during sauna treatment? Diet Health Club. [Online] July 2016. http://www.diethealthclub.com/calories-burned/calories-burnt-in-sauna.html.

39. *How the sauna affects the endocrine system.* **Kukkonen-Harjula, K and Kauppinen, K.** 4, 1988, Ann Clin Res, Vol. 20, pp. 262-266.

40. *The effect of sauna bathing on lipid profile in young, physically active, male subjects.* **Gryka, D**, et al. 4, August 27, 2014, Int J Occupational Med Environ Health., Vol. 27, pp. 608-618.

41. *Effect of a Single Finnish Sauna Session on White Blood Cell Profile and Cortisol Levels in Athletes and Non-Athletes.* **Pilch, Wanda, et al.** December 18, 2013, Journal of Human Kinetics, Vol. 39, pp. 127-135.

42. *Regular sauna bathing and the incidence of common colds.* **Ernst, E, et al.** 4, 1990, Vol. 22, pp. 225-227.

43. *Self-evaluations of factors promoting and disturbing sleep: an epidemiological survey in Finland.* **Urponen, H, et al.** 4, 1988, Vol. 26, pp. 443-450.

44. **BBC News.** Can you get the benefits of exercise by having a hot bath? BBC News. [Online] July 20, 2016. https://www.bbc.com/news/magazine-36744906.

45. *Possible use of repeated cold stress for reducing fatigue in chronic fatigue syndrome: a hypothesis.* **Shevchuk, N A.** October 24, 2007, Behav Brain Function, Vol. 3, p. 55.

46. Greenfield, Ben. Diet, Fat Loss and Performance Advice. Ben Greenfield Fitness. [Online] 2012. https://bengreenfieldfitness.com/article/fat-loss-articles/burning-more-fat-with-cold/

47. *Immune System of cold-exposed and cold-adapted humans.* **Jansky, L, et al.** 5-6, 1996, Eur J Appl Physiol Occup Physiol, Vol. 72, pp. 445-450.

48. *Energy balance and diabetes. The effects of cold exposure, exercise training, and diet composition on glucose tolerance and glucose metabolism in rat peripheral tissues.* **Bukowiecki, L J.** 4, April 1989, Can J Physiol Pharmacol, Vol. 67, pp. 382-393.

49. *Cold acclimation recruits human brown fat and increases non-shivering thermogenesis.* **Van der Lans, A A, et al.** 8, August 2013, J Clin Invest, Vol. 123, pp. 3395-3403.

50. **Odunton, Adoley and Deras, Deborah.** *Confessions of an Adrenaline Addict.* Sarasota: Healthier Living, 2012.

51. **Thoma, M V, et al.** The effect of music on the human stress response. PLOS One. [Online] August 5, 2013. https://doi.org/10.1371/journal. pone.0070156.

52. [*Histology and physiology of black skin*] *French.* **La Ruche, G and Cesarini, J P.** 8, 1992, Ann Dermatol Venereol, Vol. 119, pp. 567-574.

53. *Aging Differences in Ethnic Skin.* Vashi, **N A, Buainain De Castro Maymone, M and Kundu, R V.** 1, January 2016, J Clin Aesthet Dermatol, Vol. 9, pp. 31-38.

54. [*Skin irritation caused by propylene glycols*]. [Article in German]. **Anderson, K E and Storrs, F J.** 1, January 1982, Hautartzt, Vol. 33, pp. 12-14.

55. **The National Toxicology Program.** *Report on Carcinogens, Fourteenth Edition.* 2016.

56. *Evidence for cosmetics as a source of mineral oil contamination in women.* **Concin, N, et al.** 11, November 2011, J Womens Health (Larchmt), Vol. 20, pp. 1713-1719

57. *Comedogenicity of current therapeutic products, cosmetics, and ingredients in the rabbit ear.* **Fulton, J E Jr, Pay, S R and Fulton, J E 3rd.** 1, January 1984, J Am Acad Dermatol, Vol. 10, pp. 96-105.

58. **Phelps, Glenn and Crabtree, Steve.** Worldwide, Median Household Income About $10,000. Gallup. [Online] December 16, 2013. https://news. gallup.com/poll/166211/worldwide-median-household-income-000.aspx.

59. *Prevalence and awareness of melasma during pregnancy.* **Moin, A, Jabery, Z and Fallah, N.** 2006, Int J. Dermatol, Vol. 45, pp. 285-288.

60. *Disorders of hyperpigmentation.* **Pandya, A G and Guevara, I L.** 2000, Dermatol Clin, Vol. 18, pp. 91-98.

61. *Common dermatologic disorders in skin of color: a comparative practice survey.* *Alexis,* **A F, Sergay, A B and Taylor, S C.** 2007, Cutis, Vol. 80, pp. 387-394.

62. *Skin picking disorder.* **Grant, J E, et al.** 11, 2012, The American Journal of Psychiatry, Vol. 169, pp. 1143-1149.

63. *Update on pathological skin picking.* **Grant, J E and Odlaug, B L.** 4, 2009, Current Psychiatry Reports, Vol. 11, pp. 283-288.

64. **American Psychiatric Association.** *Diagnostic and Statistical Manual of Mental Disorders, 5th Edition: DSM-5.* Washington, DC: American Psychiatric Association, 2013.

65. **Pasternak, Annette and Fletcher, Tammy.** *Skin picking, the freedom to finally stop.* 2014.

66. *Utilizing combination therapy to optimize melasma outcomes.* **Rendon, M I.** 2004, J Drugs Dermatol, Vol. 3, pp. S27-S34.

67. *Prevalence of self-diagnosed melasma among premenopausal Latino women in Dallas and Fort Worth, Texas.* **Werlinger, K D, et al.** 2007, Arch Dermatol, Vol. 143, pp. 424-425.

68. **Food and Drug Administration.** *Proposed Rule: SPF 50 Maximum Labeled Value.* Food and Drug Administration, Department of Health and Human Services. 2011. 76FR35672.

69. The Long Way Towards the Ideal Sunscreen – *Where We Stand and What Still Needs to be Done.* **Osterwalder, U and Herzog, B.** 4, 2010, Photochemical & Photobiological Sciences, Vol. 9, pp. 470-481.

70. *Sunscreen Use and Intentional Exposure to Ultraviolet A and B Radiation: A Double Blind Randomized Trial Using Personal Dosimeters.* **Autier, P, et al.** 9, 2000, British Journal of Cancer, Vol. 83. pp. 1243-1248.

71. *Suntanning with Sunscreens: A Comparison with Sunbed Tanning.* **Diffey, B L, Osterwalder, U and Herzog, B.** 6, 2015, Photodermatology, Photoimmunology & Photomedicine, Vol. 31, pp. 307-314.

72. *The Role of Antioxidants in Photoprotection: A Critical Review.* **Chen, L, Hu, J Y and Wang, S Q.** 5, 2012, Journal of the American Academy of Dermatology, Vol. 67, pp. 1013-1024.

73. **National Toxicology Program.** *NTP Technical Report on the Photococarcinogenesis Study of Retinoic Acid and Retinyl Palmitate [CAS Nos. 302-79-4 (All-Trans-Retinoic Acid) and 79-81-2 (All-Trans-Retinyl Palmitate)] in SKH-1 Mice (Simulated Solar Light and Topical Application Study).* 2012.

74. **Bundesinstitut fur Risikobewertung.** Bundesinstitut fur Risikobewertung. [Online] January 27, 2014. www.bfr.bund.de/en/questions_ and_answers_on_the_risk_assessment_of_cosmetic_products-189042. html#topic_189052

75. **Australian Government Department of Health.** Australian Government Department of Health. [Online] January 11, 2017. www.tga.gov. au/literature-review-safety-titanium-dioxide-and-zinc-oxide-nanoparticles-sunscreens.

76. *Titanium Dioxide Nanoparticle Penetration into the Skin and Effects on HaCaT Cells.* **Crosera, M, et al.** 8, August 2015, Int J Environ Res Public Health. Vol. 12, pp. 9282-9297.

77. *ZnO particulate matter requires cell contact for toxicity in human colon cancer cells.* **Moos, P J, et al.** 4, April 19, 2010, Chem Res Toxicol, Vol. 23, pp. 733-739.

78. *Pulmonary function changes in rats after chronic and subchronic inhalation exposure to various particulate matter.* **Heinrich, U, et al.** 1989, Exp Pathol, Vol. 37, pp. 248-252.

79. *The influence of capsular extracellular polymeric substances on the interaction between TiO2 nanoparticles and planktonic bacteria.* **Hessler, C M, et al.** 15, October 1, 2012, Water Research, Vol. 46, pp. 4687-4696.

80. *Sunscreens as a Source of Hydrogen Peroxide Production in Coastal Waters.* **Sanchez-Quiles, D and Tovar-Sanchez, A.** 16, 2014, Environmental Science & Technology, Vol. 48, pp. 9037-9042.

81. *Acne in ethnic skin: special considerations for therapy.* **Callender, V D.** 2004, Dermatol Ther, Vol. 17, pp. 184-195.

82. *Exogenous ochronosis: an epidemiological study.* **Hardwick, N, et al.** 2, February 1989, Br J Dermatol, Vol. 120, pp. 229-238.

83. *Heavy metal toxicity, part I: arsenic and mercury.* **Graeme, K A and Pollack, C V.** 1998, J Emerg Med, Vol. 16, pp. 45-56.

84. *Mercury content in skin lightening creams and potential hazards to the health of Saudi women.* **Al-Saleh, I and Al-Doush, I.** 1991, J Toxicol Environ Health, Vol. 51, pp. 123-130.

85. *Perifollicular pigmentation is the first target for topical vitamin C derivative ascorbyl 2-phosphate 6-palmitate (APPS): randomized, single-blinded, placebo-controlled study.* **Inui, S and Itami, S.** 3, March 2007, J Dermatol, Vol. 34, pp. 221-223.

86. *A double-blind randomized trial of 5% ascorbic acid vs. 4% hydroquinone in melasma.* **Espinal-Perez, L E, Moncada, B and Castanedo-Cazares, J P.** 8, August 2004, Int J Dermatol, Vol. 43, pp. 604-607.

87. *Skin lightening preparations and the hydroquinone controversy.* **Draelos, Z D.** 2007, Dermatol Ther, Vol. 20, pp. 308-313.

88. *Comparison of efficacy of topical 2% liquiritin, topical 4% liquiritin and topical 4% hydroquinone in the management of melasma.* **Zubair, S and Mujtaba, G.** 2009, Journal of Pakistan Association of Dermatologists, Vol. 19, pp. 158-163.

89. *Acerola (Malpighia emarginata DC.) Juice Intake Suppresses UVB-Induced Skin Pigmentation in SMP30/GNL Knockout Hairless Mice.* **Sato, Y, et al.** 1, 2017, PLoSOne, Vol. 12.

90. *Skin-lightening effect of a polyphenol extract from Acerola (Malpighia emarginata DC.) fruit on UV-induced pigmentation.* **Hanamura, T, Uchida, E and Aoki, H.** 12, 2008, Biosci Biotechnol Biochem, Vol. 72, pp. 3211-3218.

91. *Urinary indices of hydration status.* **Armstrong, L E, et al.** 3, September 1994, Int J Sport Nutr, Vol. 4, pp. 265-279.

92. *Differential regulation of hyaluronan metabolism in the epidermal and dermal compartments of human skin by UVB irradiation.* **Averbeck, M, et al.** 3, 2007, I Invest Dermatol, Vol. 127, pp. 687-697.

93. Anti-Aging and filling efficacy of six types hyaluronic acid-based dermo-cosmetic treatment: double blind, randomized clinical trial of efficacy and safety. **Nobile, V, et al.** 4, December 2014, J Cosmet Dermatol, Vol. 13, pp. 277-287.

94. *Complications of hyaluronic acid fillers and their managements.* **Abduljabbara, M H and Basendwh, M A.** 2, July 2016, Journal of Dermatology & Dermatologic Surgery, Vol. 21, pp. 100-106.

95. *Mapping the Ligand-binding Sites and Disease-associated Mutations on the Most Abundant Protein in the Human, Type I Collagen.* **DiLullo, G A, et al.** 6, 2002, J Biol Chem, Vol. 277, pp. 4223-4231.

96. *Vitamin C Deficiency and Depletion in the United States: The Third National Health and Nutrition Examination Survey, 1988 to 1994.* **Hampl, J S, Taylor, C A and Johnston, C S.** 5, May 2004, Am J Public Health, Vol. 94, pp. 870-875.

97. *The effects of systemic hormonal replacement therapy on the skin of postmenopausal women.* **Sauerbronn, A V, et al.** 2000, Int J Gynaecol Obstet, Vol. 68, pp. 35-41.

98. *A prospective, randomized, placebo-controlled, double-blinded, and split-face clinical study on LED phototherapy for skin rejuvenation: clinical, profilometric, histologic, ultrastructural, and biochemical evaluations and comparison of three different treatment settings.* **Lee, S Y, et al.** 1, July 27, 2007, J Photochem Photobiol B, Vol. 88, pp. 51-67.

99. **Dishman, R K.** Mental Health. [book auth.] V S Seefeldt. *Physical Activity and Well Being.* Reston: American Alliance for Health, Physical Education, Recreation and Dance, 1986, pp. 303-341.

100. *Psychological Stress response following training.* **Crews, D J, et al.** 1S85, Med Sci Sport Exercise, Vol 198820Suppl.

101. **Morgan, W P.** Psychologic benefits of physical activity. [book auth.] F J Nagle and H J Montoye. *Exercise in Health and Disease.* Springfield: Charles C Thomas, 1981, pp. 299-314.

102. **Duckworth, Angela.** 2016. *Grit.* New York: Simon & Schuster.

103. *Cellular and molecular regulation of muscle regeneration.* **Charge, S B and Rudnicki, M A.** 1, January 2004, Physiol Rev, Vol. 84, pp. 209-238.

104. *Quenching Activities of Common Hydrophilic and Lipophilic Antioxidants against Singlet Oxygen Using Chemiluminescence Detection System.* **Nishida, Yasuhiro, Yamashita, Ejii and Miki, Wataru.** 2007, Carotenois Science, Vol. 11, pp. 16-20.

105. *Astaxanthin supplementation enhances adult hippocampal neurogenesis and spatial memory in mice.* **Yook, J S, et al.** 3, March 2016, Mol Nutr Food Res, Vol. 60, pp. 589-599.

106. *Astaxanthin, oxidative stress, inflammation and cardiovascular disease.* **Fassett, R G and Coobes, J S.** 4, July 2009, Future Cardiol, Vol. 5, pp. 333-342.

107. *"Effects of Astaxanthin on accommodation, critical flicker fusion, and pattern visual evoked potential in visual display terminal workers." Journal of Traditional Medicines.* **Nagaki, Y, et al.** 5, 2002, Journal of Traditional Medicines, Vol. 19, pp. 170-173.

108. *Inhibitory Effect of astaxanthin against acceleration of metastasis in the stress-loading mouse.* **Yung, s, et al.** [ed.] 428. 1997, J Nutr Food, Vol. 50, p. 423.

109. *Treatment of H. pylori infected mice with antioxidant astaxanthin reduces gastric inflammation, bacterial load and modulates cytokine release by splenocytes.* **Bennedsen, M, et al.** 1999, Immun Letters, Vol. 70, pp. 185-189.

110. *The effects of a dietary supplement containing astaxanthin on skin condition.* **Yamashita, E.** 2006, Carotenoid Science, Vol. 10, pp. 91-95.

111. *Cosmetic benefits of astaxanthin on human subjects.* **Tominaga, K, et al.** 1, 2012, Acta Biochim Pol, Vol. 59, pp. 43-47.

112. *Improvement of common cold with Pycnogenol®: a Winter registry study.* **Belcaro, G, et al.** 2014, Panminerva Med, Vol. 56, pp. 301-308.

113. *French Maritime Pine Bark Extract* (Pycnogenol®) *Effects on Human Skin: Clinical and Molecular Evidence.* **Grether-Beck, S, et al.** 1, 2016, Skin Pharmacol Physiol, Vol. 29, pp. 13-17.

114. *Pycnogenol® effects on skin elasticity and hydration coincide with increased gene expressions of collagen type I and hyaluronic acid synthase in women.* **Marini, A, et al.** 2012, Skin Pharmacol Physiol, Vol. 25, pp.

115. *Demographic Differences and Trends of Vitamin D Insufficiency in the US Population, 1988-2004.* **Ginde, A A, Liu, M C and Camargo, C A.** 6, 2009, Arch Intern Med, Vol. 169, pp. 626-632.

116. *Update in vitamin D.* **Adams, J S and Hewison, M.** 2, February 2010, J Clin Endocrinol Metab, Vol. 95, pp. 471-478.

117. *The influence of 2-dimethylaminoethanol (DMAE) on the mental and physical efficiency in man.* **Danysyz, A, Smietanski, J and Panek, W.** 4, November 1967, Act Nerv Super (Praha), Vol. 9, p. 417.

118. **Perricone, Nicholas.** 2002. *The Perricone Prescription.* New York: HarperCollins Publishers, Inc.

119. *Split face study on the cutaneous tensile effect of 2-dimethylaminoethanol (deanol) gel.* **Uhoda, I, et al.** 3, August 2002, Skin Res Technol, Vol. 8, pp. 164-167.

120. Effects of centrophenoxine on lipofuscin in the retinal pigment epithelium of old mice. **Dylewski, D P, Nandy, S and Nandy, K.** 1, 1983, Neurobio Aging, Vol. 4, pp. 89-95.

121. *Effects of centrophenoxine on lipofuscin pigments in the nervous system of old rats.* **Riga, S and Riga, D.** 2, June 7, 1974, Brain Res, Vol. 72, pp. 265-275.

122. *Topically applied vitamin C enhances the mRNA level of collagens I and III, their processing enzymes and tissue inhibitor of matrix metalloproteinase 1 in the human dermis.* **Nusgens, B V, et al.** 2001, J Invest Dermatol, Vol. 116, pp. 853-849.

123. *Green tea EGCG, T cells, and T cell-mediated autoimmune diseases.* **Wu, D, Wang, J P and Meydani, S N.** 1, 2012, Molecular Aspects of Medicine, Vol. 33, pp. 107-118.

124. Green tea polyphenols avert chronic inflammation-induced myocardial fibrosis of female rats. **Shen, C L, et al.** 7, 2011, Inflammation Research, Vol. 60, pp. 665-672.

125. *Green tea catechin extract in intervention of chronic breast cell carcinogenesis induced by environmental carcinogens.* **Rathore, K and Wang, H-CR.** 3, 2012, Molecular carcinogenesis, Vol. 51, pp. 280-289.

126. *Green tea prevents non-melanoma skin cancer by enhancing DNA repair.* **Kativar, S K.** 2, April 15, 2011, Arch Biochem Biophys, Vol. 508, pp. 152-158.

127. *Green tea extract protects human skin fibroblasts from reactive oxygen species induced necrosis.* **Silverberg, J I, et al.** 10, 2011, Journal of Drugs in Dermatology, Vol. 10, pp. 1096-1101.

128. *Anti-angiogenic effects of epigallocatechin-3-gallate in human skin.* **Domingo, D S, et al.** 7, 2010, International Journal of Clinical and Experimental Pathology, Vol. 3, pp. 705-709.

129. *Photoprotective effects of a formulation containing tannase-converted green tea extract against UVB-induced oxidative stress in hairless mice.* **Hong, Y-H, et al.** 1, 2012, Applied Biochemistry and Biotechnology, Vol. 166, pp. 165-175.

130. *Green tea catechins reduce invasive potential of human melanoma cells by targeting COX-2, PGE2 receptors and epithelial-to-mesenchymal transition.* **Singh, T and Katiyar, S K**. 10, 2011, PLoS ONE, Vol. 6, p. e25224.

131. *Inhibition of melanoma growth and metastasis by combination with (-)-epigallocatechin-3-gallate and dacarbazine in mice.* **Liu, J D, et al,** 4, 2001, Journal of Cellular Biochemistry, Vol. 83, pp. 631-642.

132. *The 500 Dalton rule for the skin penetration of chemical compounds and drugs.* **Bos, J D and Meinardi, M M.** 3, June 2000, Exp Dermatol, Vol. 9, pp. 165-169.

133. *Oral supplementation of specific collagen peptides has beneficial effects on human skin physiology: a double-blind, placebo-controlled study.* **Proksch, E, et al.** 1, 2014, Skin Pharmacol Physiol, Vol. 27, pp. 47-55.

134. *Oral Administration of Polymer Hyaluronic Acid Alleviates Symptoms of Knee Osteoarthritis: A Double-Blind, Placebo-Controlled Study over a 12-Month Period.* **Tashiro, T, et al.** 2012, Scientific World Journal, Vol. 167928.

135. *Clinical study shows hyaluronic acid in BioCell Collagen II® found to have significant absorption and bioavailability.* **Judy, William.** 2004.

136. **Sardi, Bill.** *How to Live to be 100 Years Without Growing Old.* s.l.: Here and Now Books, 2002.

137. *Hyaluronan Exists in the Normal Stratum Corneum.* **Sakai, S, et al.** 6, 2000, Journal of Investigative Dermatology, Vol. 114, pp. 1184-1187.

138. *Oral Intake of a Liquid High-Molecular-Weight Hyaluronan Associated with Relief of Chronic Pain and Reduced Use of Pain Medication: Results of a Randomized, Placebo-Controlled Double-Blind Pilot Study.* **Jensen, G S, et al.** 1, January, 2015, Med Food, Vol. 18, pp. 95-101.

139. **Physicians Desk Reference, Inc.** *Physicians Desk Reference (PDR) for Nutritional Supplements 1st ed.* Montvale: Physicians Desk Reference Inc., 2001.

140. *"Dehydroepiandrosterone and its metabolites: differential effects on androgen receptor trafficking and transcriptional activity".* **Mo, Q, Lu, S F and Simon, N G.** 1, April 2006, The Journal of Stroid Biochemistry and Molecular Biology, Vol. 99, pp. 50-58.

141. **Scott, T.** *Concise Encyclopedia Biology.* s.l.: Walter du Gruyter, 1996.

142. *Dehydroepiandrosterone (DHEA), DHEA sulfate, and aging: contribution of the DHEAge Study to a sociobiomedical issue.* **Baulieu, E E, et al.** 8, April 11, 2000, Proc National Academy Science U S A, Vol. 97, pp. 4279-4284.

143. *DHEA, important source of sex steroids in men and even more in women.* **Labrie, F.** 2010, Prog Brain Res, Vol. 182, pp. 182-197.

144. *DHEA, DHEA-S and cortisol responses to acute exercise in older adults in relation to exercise training status and sex.* **Heaney, J L J, Carroll, D and Phillips, A C.** 2, April 2013, Age (Dordr), Vol. 25, pp. 395-405.

145. *Acute hormonal responses of a high impact physical exercise session in early postmenopausal women.* **Kemmler, W, et al.** 1-2, September 2003, European Journal of Applied Physiology, Vol. 90, pp. 199-209.

146. **Muller, R A and Muller, E A.** Air Pollution and Cigarette Equivalence. *Berkely Earth.* [Online] httP://berkeleyearth.org/air-pollution-and-cigaretter-equivalence/.

147. *Prevalence, severity and severity risk factors of acne in high school pupils: A community-based study.* **Ghodsi, S Z, Orawa H and Zouboulis, C C.** 9, September 2009, J Invest Dermatol, Vol. 129, pp. 2136-2141.

148. *Persistent acne in women: implications for the patient and for therapy.* **Williams, C and Layton, A M.** 2006, Am J Clin Dermatol, Vol. 7, pp. 281-290.

149. *Post-adolescent acne: a review of clinical features.* **Goulden, V, Clark, S M and Cunliffe, W J.** 1997, Br J Dermatol, Vol. 136, pp. 66-70.

150. *Acne and smoking.* **Capitanio, B, et al.** 3, May-June 2009, Dermatoendocrinol, Vol. 1, pp. 129-135.

151. *Nicotine effects on the skin: are they positive or negative?* **Misery, L.** 2004, Exp Dermatol, Vol. 13, pp. 665-670.

152. *Cigarette smoking associated with premature facial wrinkling: image analysis of facial skin replicas.* **Koh, J, et al.** 2002, Int J Dermatol, Vol. 41, pp. 21-27.

153. *Cigarette smoke-induced lipid peroxidation in human skin and its inhibition by topically applied antioxidants.* **Pelle, E, et al.** 2002, Skin Pharmacol Appl Skin Physiol, Vol. 15, pp. 63-68.

154. *The Organization of Human Epidermis: Functional Epidermal Units and Phi Proportionality.* **Hoath, S B and Leahy, D G.** 6, December 2003, Journal of Investigative Dermatology, Vol. 121, pp. 1440-1446.

155. *Making An Epidermis.* **Koster, Maranke.** July 2009, Ann N Y Acad Sci, Vol. 1170, pp. 7-10.

156. **American Contact Dermatitis Society**. Allergen of the Year. *American Contact Dermatitis Society.* [Online] 2013. www.contactderm.org/i4a/pages/index.cfm?pageid=3467.

157. *The evaluation of aluminum oxide crystal microdermabrasion for photodamage.* **Tan, M H, et al.** 11, November 2001, Dermatol Surg, Vol. 27, pp. 943-949.

158. *Bromelain's activity and potential as an anti-cancer agent: Current evidence and perspectives.* **Chobotova, K, Vernallis, A B and Majid, F A**. 2, 2010, Cancer Letters, Vol. 290, pp. 148-156.

159. *A theory for the mechanism of action of the alpha-hydroxy acids applied to the skin.* **Wang, X.** 5, November 1999, Med Hypotheses, Vol. 53, pp. 380-382.

160. *Photoprotective Potential of Glycolic Acid by Reducing NLRC4 and AIM2 Inflammasome Complex Proteins in UVB Radiation-Induced Normal Human Epidermal Keratinocytes and Mice.* **Hung, S J, et al.** 2, February 2017, DNA Cell Biol, Vol. 36, pp. 177-187.

161. *The Effects of Topically Applied Glycolic Acid and Salicylic Acid on Ultraviolet Radiation-Induced Erythema, DNA Damage and Sunburn Cell Formation in Human Skin.* **Kornhauser, A, et al.** 1, July 2009, J Dermatol Sci, Vol. 55, pp. 10-17.

162. *Salicylate intoxication after use of topical salicylic acid ointment by a patient with psoriasis.* **Pec, J, et al.** 4, October 1992, Cutis, Vol. 50, pp. 307-309.

163. *Acute perceptive hearing loss and metabolic acidosis as complications of the topical treatment of psoriasis with salicylic acid-containing ointment]. [Article in Dutch].* **Jongevos, S F, et al.** 43, October 25, 1997, Ned Tijdschr Geneeskd, Vol. 141, pp. 2075-2079.

164. *The life and Times of the LED - a 100-year history.* **Zheludev, Nikolay.** 4, April 2007, Nature Photonics: Nature Publishing Group, Vol. 1, pp. 189-192.

165. *Light-emitting diodes (LEDs) in dermatology.* **Barolet, D B** 2008, Semin Cutan Med Surg, Vol. 27, pp. 227-238.

166. *Regulation of skin collagen metabolism in vitro using a pulsed 660 nm LED light source: clinical correlation with a single-blinded study.* **Barolet, D, et al.** 2009, J Invest Dermatol, Vol. 129, pp. 2751-2759.

167. *Immunohistochemical expression of matrix metalloproteinases in photodamaged skin by photodynamic therapy.* **Almeida Issa, M C, et al**. 2009, Br J Dermatol, Vol. 161, pp. 647-653.

168. *Red light-emitting diode (LED) therapy accelerates wound healing post-blepharoplasty and periocular laser ablative resurfacing.* **Trelles, M A and Allones, I.** 1, April 2006, J Cosmet Laser Ther, Vol. 8, pp. 39-42.

169. *Er: YAG laser ablation of plantar verrucae with red LED therapy-assisted healing.* **Trelles, M A, Allones, I and Mayo, E.** 4, August 2006, Photomed Laser Surg, Vol. 24, pp. 494-498.

170. *Light-emitting Diodes. A Brief Review and Clinical Experience.* **Opel, D R, et al.** 6, June 2015, J Clin Aesthet Dermatol, Vol. 8, pp. 36-44.

171. *Light-emitting diode 415nm in the treatment of inflammatory acne: an open-label, multicentric, pilot investigation.* **Tremblay, J F, et al.** 2006, J Gosmet Laser Ther, Vol. 8, pp.31-33.

172. *Clinical efficacy of home-use blue-light therapy for mild-to-moderate acne.* **Gold, M H, Sensing, W and Biron, J A.** 2011, J Gosmet Laser Ther, Vol. 13, pp. 308-314.

173. *Evaluation of self-treatment of mild-to-moderate facial acne with a blue light treatment system.* **Wheeland, R G and Dhawan, S.** 2011, J Drugs Dermatol, Vol. 10, pp. 596-602.

174. *Augmentation of wound healing using monochromatic infrared energy: exploration of a new technology for wound management.* **Horwitz, L R, Burke, T J and Carnegie, D.** 1999, Adv Wound Care, Vol. 12, pp. 35-40.

175. *New treatment of cellulite with infrared-LED illumination applied during high-intensity treadmill training.* **Paolillo, F R, et al.** 2011, J Gosmet Laser Ther, Vol. 13, pp. 166-171.

176. *Antiphotoaging effects of light-emitting diode irradiation on narrow-band ultraviolet B-exposed cultured human skin cells.* **Tian, Y S, Kim, N H and Lee, A Y.** 10, October 2012, Dermatol Surg, Vol. 38, pp. 1695-1703.

177. *Perspectives on transdermal ultrasound mediated drug delivery.* **Smith, N B.** 4, December 2007, Int J Nanomedicine, Vol. 2, pp. 585-594.

ABOUT THE BRUTALLY HONEST AUTHORS

Tanis Rhines is a scientist turned esthetician exposing the truth about all things' beauty. She is a prolific writer tackling tough topics; often in a humorous, but always in an honest way. She lives with her cichlid, Creamsicle, at the sunny tip of Florida and spends most of her time body surfing, busting myths and bicycling.

Neddy Rodriguez is a makeup artist turned passionate esthetician with an eye for honesty. She curates esthetic master classes, fostering growth in colleagues while building community. She lives in LA where she rocks her Cuban and Puerto Rican genes at salsa venues and enjoys spending time with her family, friends, and adorable doggie, Ralphie. Woof!

You can meet them in person by attending one of their classes or presentations, chat them up on social media, or just crack up at their postings on the following Ask the Estheticians sites:

facebook.com/asktheestheticians

twitter.com/AskTheEsthes

instagram.com/asktheestheticians

pinterest.com/asktheestheticians

INDEX

A

Acerola, 148

Acne, 2, 9, 28, 30-32, 34-37, 43-46,
54-57, 62, 64, 69, 71, 79, 101,
102, 207, 208, 235, 236, 245-
248, 259, 260, 273-275

Adrenal fatigue, 56, 79

Alcohol, 184-186

Almond oil, 22, 87

Aloe, 97

Alpha hydroxy acid, 102, 144, 231

Androgens, 46, 53-55, 201

Antioxidants, 133, 187, 188, 208, 210

Anti-pollution, 194, 208

Arbutin, 146, 148

Ascorbic acid (also see vitamin C),
101, 147, 193, 194, 231

Astaxanthin, 187-189

Atrazine, 60

B

Benzaldehyde, 21

Beta hydroxy acid, 102, 196, 234, 235

Biotin, 199, 200

Birth control pill, 43, 64

Botox, 154, 155, 159, 160, 163,
165-167

BPA, 60

C

Carbohydrate, 30, 32, 33, 43, 56

Ceramides, 86, 261, 262

Chemical peel, 159, 228-231, 237, 265

Chronoaging, 161

Circulation, 70, 189, 208, 246, 247

Citric acid, 231

Cleanser, 10, 12-15, 22, 23, 57, 86, 87

Cocaine, 187

Coconut oil, 22, 87, 129, 197

Collagen, 9, 30, 59, 101, 141, 154,
160, 167-172, 180, 190, 193-
199, 208, 223, 229, 232, 237,

243, 245, 246, 248, 267, 274, 280-283

Comedogenic, 20-22, 93, 100, 101, 103, 104, 219

COVID, 256, 257, 259-261, 263-265, 267-269

Cryotherapy, 72-74, 144

D

D&C Red, 22

Dairy, 28, 34-37, 47, 61

Dehydration, 161, 217

Dermcidin, 69, 70

Dermaplaning, 266, 267

Dermatitis, 21, 98, 101, 142, 220, 260

Dermis, 59, 84, 129, 161, 162, 215

DHEA, 53, 54, 154, 200-203

Diabetes, 43, 49, 198, 206

Dioxin, 60, 61

DMAE, 192, 193

E

Eczema, 36, 79, 98, 120, 220

Elasticity, 59, 102, 160, 161, 169-171, 188, 193, 197, 199, 236

Elastin, 141, 169-171, 208, 229, 232, 237, 267

Endosulfan, 61

Enzymes, 36, 142, 168, 194, 198, 214, 222, 223

Epidermis, 59, 96, 97, 100, 160, 169, 194, 195, 215-217, 222, 231, 235, 250

Essential oil, 62-64, 221

Estrogen, 43, 46, 54-64, 132, 161, 201, 202

Ethylhexyl palmitate, 22

Excoriation disorder(ED), 121

Exercise, 18, 31, 37, 43, 46, 56, 57, 66, 68, 71, 72, 79, 85, 154, 171, 176-181, 202, 203, 233, 245

Exfoliation, 44, 102, 114, 141, 143, 214, 215, 218, 219, 221-224, 229, 232, 233, 266

Extraction, 69, 85, 154, 265

F

Fillers, 159, 161-164

Folliculitis, 234

Free radicals, 46, 133, 187, 223

G

Glutathione, 171, 179

Glycerin, 96, 97

Glycolic acid, 144, 196, 223, 231-234

Greasy food, 33, 37

Green algae, 187, 188

Green tea, 14, 194, 210

H

Heroin, 186

Hormonal breakouts, 46, 53-57, 61, 62, 64-66

Hormone replacement therapy (HRT), 53, 64, 65, 123, 161, 171

CPSIA information can be obtained
at www.ICGtesting.com
Printed in the USA
JSHW050140080722
27700JS00005B/140